SIMPLE SUPERFOOD SMOOTHIES

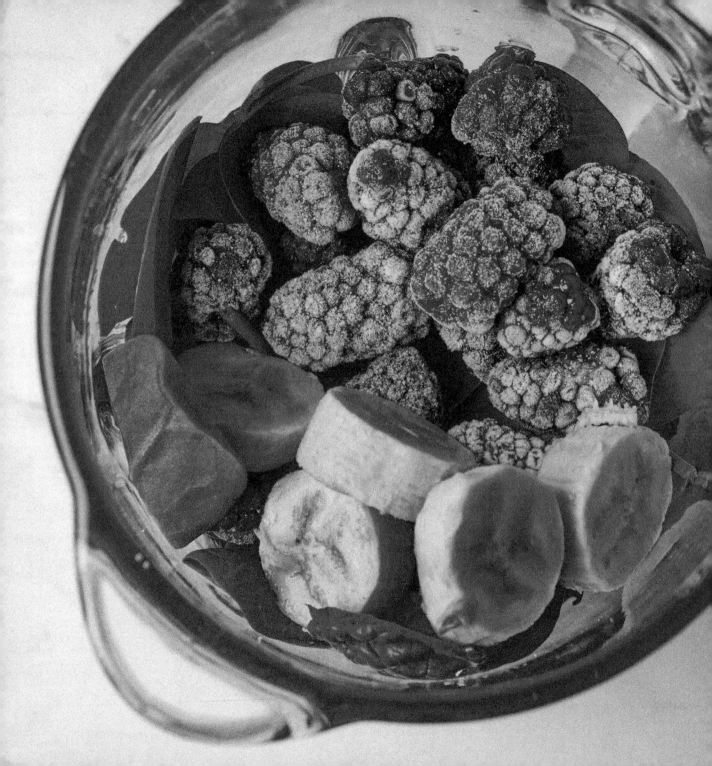

Simple
SUPERFOOD
SMOOTHIES

A Smoothie Recipe Book
to Supercharge Your Health

SONDI BRUNER

PHOTOGRAPHY BY EVI ABELER

ROCKRIDGE
PRESS

For my husband

Interior and Cover Designer: Michael Cook
Photo Art Director: Sue Smith
Editor: Crystal Nero
Production Editor: Ashley Polikoff
Photography © 2019 Evi Abeler. Food styling by Albane Sharrard.
Author photo: Stephanie Chan/The Pauhaus

ISBN: Print 978-1-64152-587-9 | eBook 978-1-64152-588-6

Contents

Introduction

Smoothies always provide a quick and convenient meal in my household. In fact, it's hard to remember a time when they weren't a part of my life, but the truth is I didn't discover the beauty of the smoothie until I neared my mid-twenties. Until that point, I had never even seen a person consume a smoothie. But on taking my first sip, I was instantly hooked on the burst of flavor and intensity.

At first, I relied on smoothies mainly for their taste. I didn't pay much attention to their health benefits or prepare them myself—I just purchased them from smoothie bars. Later, in 2006, eight years after being diagnosed with Crohn's disease (an autoimmune digestive disorder), I realized I needed to take control of my health and focus on consuming foods that would help ease my symptoms, address inflammation, and boost immunity. My diet and lifestyle at the time were simply not supportive of digestive health. This led to little appetite and difficulty eating, constant bloating and gassiness, countless hours in the bathroom, and severe anemia. Essentially, my quality of life was poor, and if I wanted to live vibrantly, I had to make changes.

I began cooking almost everything from scratch, a big adjustment as I was accustomed to buying many packaged items. Soon I was learning how to bake my own crackers and whip up condiments, and I invested in a cheap blender so I could make smoothies, dips, and sauces at home.

Smoothies are beneficial to a wide range of health conditions, but for me they were life-changing, because I could pack many more nutrient-dense ingredients into a single glass than I could ever consume in one sitting if I left those foods in their whole forms. Smoothies made it easier for me to eat without pain or discomfort and take in the nutrients I was missing. They were also dead simple to blend, which enabled me to make smoothies a habit.

Once I started nutrition school and learned about the amazing benefits of superfoods, I began honing my smoothie techniques with both whole foods and superfood powders. Here's where my smoothies veered out of control: They became time-consuming, complicated (I would often add 12 to 15 ingredients to the blender, several of which were concentrated powders), and a heck of a lot more expensive. While some ingredients are worth the money if you are targeting a specific health issue or have a nutrient deficiency, it was not sustainable for me to keep creating these superfood monsters. And so, after about a year, I returned to the basics: blending fruit, veggies, nuts, seeds, spices, herbs, and liquids to make delicious, health-building smoothies.

Superfoods are all around us—you can conveniently find them at your local grocery store without breaking the bank. With this book, it's my goal to help you discover the benefits of everyday ingredients and create deliciously simple smoothies that will bring you good health. You deserve it!

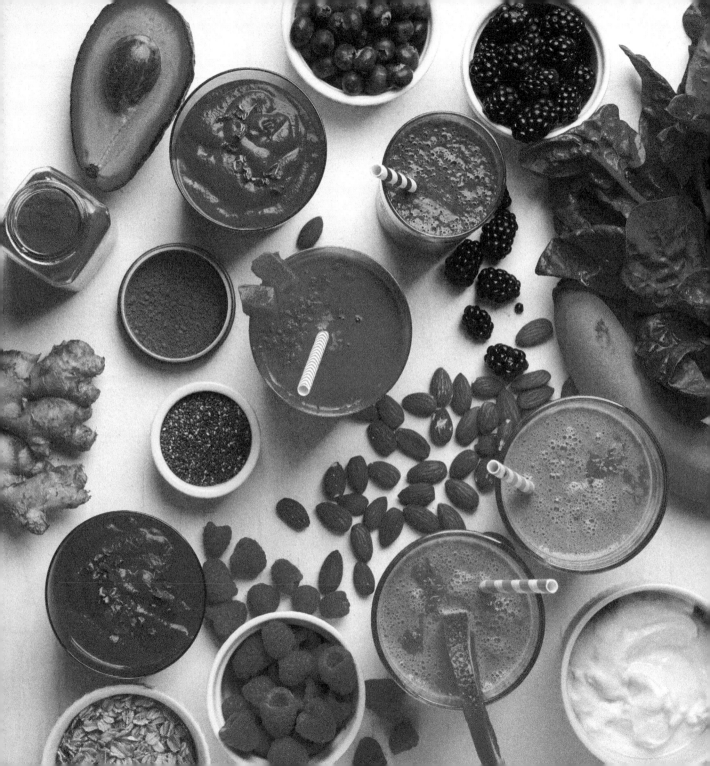

Supercharge Your Health with Superfood Smoothies

Amid our modern lives, it can be challenging to prioritize our health. Some view busyness as a status symbol or a source of pride, but for many of us, it's not always possible to tear up the to-do list or escape to a rustic, Wi-Fi–free cabin in the mountains for a week. Between work, family, friends, hobbies, volunteering, and exercise, it can be difficult to find the time to eat, much less cook! Still, neglecting our health in the present can lead to serious, chronic consequences in the future—and this may compromise our ability to take care of ourselves and those important to us. We can't be there for those we love if we are too sick to enjoy the precious time we have.

Enter the smoothie: a convenient, affordable, efficient way to facilitate health. Smoothies require no cooking, so you can prep or blend them in batches ahead of time, and you can even take one with you on the go. If you're curious about how you can use specific superfoods to strategically enhance the health benefits of your smoothies, the recipes here will help you explore beneficial ingredients and how you can make them taste wonderful, too.

Why Superfoods?

If you've watched television or picked up a magazine or newspaper in the last couple of decades, you've probably heard the word "superfood." Often, these news stories or features tout a trendy ingredient that is the best or latest thing you must include in your diet.

There isn't a scientific or legal definition for the word superfood, so there isn't a conclusive and official meaning—it depends on who you ask. The food industry is criticized for exploiting superfoods as a marketing tactic to sell products, and to some extent, this critique is true: No single ingredient will magically and instantly improve your health, and there are consumers who are lulled by label claims, even if a product contains other harmful ingredients like added sugars or known endocrine disruptors. Some foods are advertised as the exclusive source of rare and special nutrients, yet nature tends to have redundancies. If you can't afford a powder of an omega-3–rich superfood, rest assured you will be able to find those healthy fats elsewhere.

Still, it's fair to describe superfoods as nutrient-dense ingredients that are beneficial to our health. This is a broad definition, but one I like because it includes simple and accessible ingredients. Simply put, superfoods contain macronutrients, vitamins, minerals, antioxidants, and other compounds that affect our health. You don't need to venture to the ends of the Earth for expensive foods—superfood ingredients are all around us. We just need to appreciate these everyday ingredients for their valuable attributes. For example, a modest clove of garlic packs a large nutritional punch that benefits immunity and cardiovascular health. Swathes of ingredients, including vegetables, fruits, nuts, seeds, beans, legumes, fish, eggs, poultry, and even red meat, have unique and helpful compounds.

Some scientific literature alludes to "functional foods," roughly defined as foods that may improve health or prevent disease. Investigations into specific superfoods—fruits and vegetables in particular—have found that these ingredients can reduce our risk of chronic diseases such as cancer, heart disease, obesity, and diabetes, as well as contain nutrients that reduce inflammation, boost immunity, and protect gut health.

Your superfood smoothie journey can begin by using basics that are easily accessible at your local grocer. You don't need to drop a load of cash on pricey powders—one ingredient isn't going to make or break your health. Good health builds with every choice you make, and all of the everyday, nutritious ingredients add up!

The Big 15

I could highlight dozens of foods to use in smoothies, but in the interest of keeping the recipes simple and straightforward, I've selected 15 key superfoods to get you started.

This book is divided into two parts: The first features superfood basics, ingredients that function as the base of your smoothies, while the second section focuses on ingredients that work best as superfood "boosts," those you only use in small amounts for their health benefits and contribution to flavor.

The first section will feature:

- **Common Berries**
- **Bananas**
- **Common Nuts and Seeds**
- **Dark Leafy Greens**
- **Yogurt and Kefir**
- **Avocado**
- **Beets**
- **Oats**

The second section will feature:

- **Cinnamon**
- **Cacao/Cocoa**
- **Ginger**
- **Turmeric**
- **Green Tea and Matcha**
- **Pomegranate and Acai**
- **Chia Seeds**

These 15 foods are all high in key nutrients, the specifics of which you will learn more about in later chapters. Readily available in most grocery stores, these ingredients are affordable and easy to store in your pantry, refrigerator, or freezer, and they impart great flavor to smoothies. You may already have some of these at home,

making it even easier for you to begin without delay (or excuses!).

With each chapter, you will learn how to effectively use these ingredients to build smoothies that are nutritionally balanced, tasty, satiating, and well-textured.

Getting Started

Whether you're a smoothie newbie or stuck in a smoothie rut, the next few sections offer tips and advice to help you make your superfood smoothies a success. You'll discover the key components essential to every smoothie, handy tools of the trade, smoothie troubleshooting, best practices for storing and shopping for superfoods, and more.

Smoothie Basics

Whether you intend for your smoothie to be consumed as a meal or a snack, always aim to incorporate the following components:

- **Fiber**
- **Protein**
- **Fat**
- **Liquid**

The first three elements will amp up the staying power of your smoothie, helping you feel satisfied and satiated, as well as provide you with the valuable macronutrients you need throughout the day. Fruits, vegetables, nuts, and seeds are all sources of fiber. Nuts and seeds (as well as their butters) are also good sources of protein and fat. Additional sources of protein include protein powders or beans (yes, beans!), and remember that veggies and fruits contain small amounts of protein, too. You can find healthy fats in oils (coconut, flax, hemp, chia, olive), as well as in ghee and nut/seed milks.

The final component, liquid, will help your smoothie blend easily and provide you with hydration for digestion, circulation, skin health, and nutrient absorption, while flushing out waste. Water is the easiest, cheapest, and most convenient option, but you can also use nut/seed milk, coconut water, or 100 percent fruit juice.

Smoothie Blending Tips

Various experts and chefs have their favorite methods for the best way to layer a smoothie, and I have mine, too. Generally, I add ingredients to the blender in the following order:

1. **Liquids (this provides a vortex so the rest of the ingredients get sucked into the blades)**
2. **Greens, veggies, and herbs, if used in large amounts**
3. **Fruit**
4. **Nuts/seeds/nut butters/yogurt**
5. **Spices and powders**

However, there may be instances where you'd want to add the spices and powders after the liquid: For example, if you are including a protein powder, it may not fully dissolve if it's added on top of everything. It also depends on what kind of machine you own and the size of the container. If you have a regular blender, you may need to blend the liquids with the greens and veggies first before adding the remaining ingredients to ensure that everything mixes evenly (and that you don't end up with any large veggie chunks).

No matter your blender, I recommend starting on the slowest speed so ingredients can begin to integrate, and then gradually increasing the speed. If you go from "off" to "high" right away, your ingredients will likely fly around the blender and then get stuck beneath the blades.

I'm not a fan of adding ice to smoothies, as it can water down the taste and be challenging for some machines to blend smoothly. I may include it if the other ingredients are cool or at room temperature and I'm aiming for a slushier texture.

If you'd like to experiment, try ice in crushed form or small cubes for easier blending rather than large cubes.

As you practice your smoothie-making skills, you'll get to know the intricacies of your blender and what works best for you. I don't think there is a definitive "right" way to blend a smoothie, so don't get too caught up in the order of blending. Follow your instincts, which you will hone as you go.

Smoothie Prep Tips

Smoothies are quick to prepare, but sometimes, even with the best of intentions, we run out of time in the morning or life simply gets in the way. The solution? Smoothie kits! These allow you to batch prep ingredients so your smoothie can be ready in seconds. Here's how you do it:

1. Wash, prep, and measure out ingredients for your smoothies (except for the liquid).
2. Put the ingredients in a baggie or jar, seal, and label with the smoothie name.
3. When you are ready to sip, pour the liquid into the blender, dump in the contents of the bag or jar, and blend.

The number of smoothie kits you create will depend on your freezer space, but you can easily prep your smoothies for the workweek (five kits) as a good start.

Another option is to fully blend the smoothie and then freeze it. Store each one in a mason jar or another freezer-safe cup, ensuring you leave at least an inch of headspace to allow for expansion. Remember you will need time for the smoothie to defrost, which can take from 12 to 14 hours in the refrigerator, so plan accordingly if you want to drink your smoothie first thing in the morning. At room temperature, a smoothie will take from 2 to 3 hours to thaw. This is a good option if you want to grab it from the freezer in the morning and consume it later as a snack or at lunch.

Troubleshooting Your Smoothie

Despite their simplicity, superfood smoothies can have some common pitfalls. When you're working with limited ingredients and time, a chalky or slimy smoothie can really turn you off. Let's chat about some common smoothie problems and how you can resolve them.

Problem: Your smoothie is too tart/sour.
Solution: Add a natural sweetener such as maple syrup, honey, coconut sugar, dates, raisins, or stevia.

Equipment + Tools for Superfood Smoothies

The essential tool for making superfood smoothies is a blender. You have several blender options to choose from:

High-Speed Blender. This type of machine is my personal favorite. I hemmed and hawed about buying one for over a year, and my only regret is that I didn't purchase it sooner. High-speeds make smoothies very smooth and creamy, are very fast, and can be used for many other recipes in the kitchen. It's not unusual for me to use my high-speed blender several times a day. They are pricey, but you can look for refurbished ones online that cost less.

Regular Blender. A normal countertop blender will do a great job, particularly if you are new to making smoothies and aren't sure you want to make a huge investment. Some blenders will have a smoothie button that is more effective at crushing ice and other tough ingredients. You may find you need to add a little more liquid to bring your smoothie together in a regular blender as opposed to a high-speed, and your smoothie won't be quite as velvety smooth. However, your result will still be delicious!

Single-Serve Blender. This type of blender is convenient because you can blend your smoothie, then remove the jar and use it as a glass (it also comes with a lid if you want to take it with you). These are typically quite powerful, and as a bonus, there is less cleanup. The downside is you can only make one serving at a time.

Aside from a blender, you'll need minimal equipment: Measuring cups and spoons are helpful, along with a tamper to help push ingredients toward the blades for smooth blending—many blenders come with one.

Lastly, a helpful (but not essential) smoothie accessory is a glass straw. I like using glass straws because they are reusable, durable, dishwasher-safe, and you can see through them, so you know they are clean. Stainless steel straws are also a good option.

Start off with ½ teaspoon, and add more as needed. A quarter of a banana helps, too, or a sweet spice such as ground cinnamon.

Problem: Your smoothie is too sweet.
Solution: Add freshly squeezed lemon or lime juice. In the future, scale back on the very sweet fruits (like banana, mango, figs, and grapes) to start, and then add more if needed.

Problem: Your smoothie is too thin.
Solution: Add frozen fruit, avocado, chia seeds, or flaxseed (these "gel" up in water), cooked pumpkin/sweet potato purée, frozen cauliflower, yogurt, nut butter, or smoothie cubes from leftover smoothies (see Made Too Much?, page xvii).

Problem: Your smoothie is too thick.
Solution: Thin with water, nondairy milk, or 100 percent juice. Add a little at a time, or you may overshoot and end up with a smoothie that's too thin! Another option is to use fresh fruit instead of frozen, or fruits with high water content such as melons, oranges, grapes, or cucumber.

Problem: Your smoothie is too chunky/not blending properly.
Solution: Cut vegetables and fruits into smaller pieces so they blend more easily, blending your greens with liquids first. Remember to start at a low speed and gradually increase to higher speeds. Also be sure to stop the blender at intervals if ingredients are getting stuck, and stir the mixture. You may also need to add more liquid.

Problem: Your smoothie tastes too "green."
Solution: No one really wants to drink a salad. Try adding half a frozen banana, berries, a date, maple syrup, honey, mango, pineapple, 100 percent juice, or coconut milk (don't add all of these at once, but choose one or two for troubleshooting). Keep in mind that some greens are quite bitter when blended in smoothies, like dandelion or collards. You can absolutely build up your tolerance for these, but start small. Baby greens, which are milder in flavor, are also helpful.

Problem: Your smoothie separates.
Solution: Give it a quick shake or stir.

Problem: Your smoothie is stringy.
Solution: Some vegetables like celery, ginger, and stems of greens don't blend entirely if your machine isn't strong enough. To eliminate the unblended bits, strain your entire smoothie or blend the stringier items with water first, strain, and then proceed with the rest of the ingredients.

Problem: Your smoothie is dull or doesn't really taste like anything.
Solution: Only use the recipes in this book—just kidding. We all have different palates, and sometimes a smoothie will taste only so-so to you. First, choose high-quality ingredients that are in season or were flash frozen when they were in season (after all, a tasteless melon in January won't suddenly taste more intensely watermelony just because you put it in your smoothie). Improve smoothie flavors with herbs and spices (you'll find several options in part 2 of this book). Another game changer is a pinch of

sea salt: While we are accustomed to using salt in savory dishes or baked goods, remember that salt is a flavor enhancer and a worthwhile addition to all smoothies.

Building Your Superfood Stash

Superfood smoothies are simple to whip up at a moment's notice if you have a well-stocked pantry, refrigerator, and freezer. Some superfood ingredients won't need much storage space (such as dried spices), while others may require more prep and room in your refrigerator or freezer. Building a good pantry takes time, so start with one item at a time—perhaps the ingredients or flavors you enjoy the most.

As with other types of recipes, a tasty smoothie begins with quality ingredients. You'll learn more about what to look for in each smoothie chapter, but overall, it's a good rule of thumb to purchase the best quality you can find and afford. I like to buy local, organic ingredients when possible for my health and the health of the planet. A review of over 300 studies of organic crops in the *British Journal of Nutrition* concluded that organics contain more antioxidants and fewer pesticides and

Made Too Much?

Don't toss extras away!

- If your eyes were bigger than your stomach and there is enough left over for a small serving, seal your smoothie in a jar and store in the refrigerator. Drink within 24 hours. If you won't be drinking it that soon, freeze in a freezer-safe jar (be sure to leave an inch of space at the top to allow for expansion).
- If there is a bit left over, but not quite a full serving, pour into ice cube trays and freeze for use in future smoothies.
- If you have children and there is enough to fill a small glass, then share!
- Make fruit leather: Spread leftover smoothie on a parchment-lined baking sheet, and dehydrate in the oven at its lowest temperature until dry.
- Use leftovers in baked goods like muffins, cookies, breads, and brownies. This tends to work better with smoothies that are fruitier and less green.

heavy metals, while another study in the same journal noted organic milk has more omega-3 fatty acids (important for skin health, digestion, and cognition) and a healthier fat profile than conventional milk. Check out the Dirty Dozen and the Clean Fifteen (see page 197), which lists the fruits and vegetables with the most and least pesticide residues. It's a wonderful guide to help you prioritize which ingredients to buy organic.

Local ingredients are also a fabulous option as produce loses nutritional value as soon as it is plucked from the ground or picked from a bush or tree. By purchasing fresh, local ingredients, you cut down the travel time from farm to plate, and your food will retain more nutrients and flavor. Let's look at some specific tips for shopping and storing the Big 15 superfoods highlighted in this book.

Avocado: Picking the perfect avocado can be tricky. Avocados will ripen after harvest and darken as they do. If the avocados in the store look ripe, give them a gentle squeeze—they should yield to pressure, but not collapse under your fingers. Another trick is to check under the stem at the top: If it's green underneath, it's still good.

If it's brown/black, the avocado is over-ripe. I'm generally not a fan of freezing avocados because the texture becomes odd when they thaw. But if you toss your frozen avocado straight into a smoothie, this won't be an issue.

Bananas: Some grocery stores will save brown bananas for customers who like to bake or make smoothies. Speak to your produce manager about this, and you'll probably get a good deal on them. Store in a dark cupboard until ripe (i.e., with many brown spots). Slice, place on a parchment-lined baking sheet, freeze, and then store in a freezer-safe container.

Beets: Look for smooth, firm beets with no blemishes or shriveled bits. If the beet greens are still attached, save them to use in smoothies or stir-fries. Store in the crisper.

Cacao/Cocoa: Cacao powder has either been minimally heated or is still raw, while cocoa is roasted. The former tends to be more bitter, though the variety of cocoa bean also plays a role. Store in the pantry.

Chia Seeds: Buy whole chia seeds instead of ground. Chia contains delicate fats that are susceptible to heat, light, and air, and the grinding process will oxidize those fats and increase their potential for becoming rancid. Store in the refrigerator.

Cinnamon: Purchase ground in small amounts rather than bulk for optimum freshness. Store in the pantry.

Common Berries: You can purchase numerous varieties of berries in a single clamshell or bag, or you might buy a bag of mixed berries. If buying fresh, look for berries that are firm (not mushy), and be sure to check at the bottom of the container for any mold. Store in the freezer.

Common Nuts and Seeds: If buying from grocery bulk bins, purchase from stores that have a high turnover to obtain the freshest nuts (you don't want to scoop from a bin where almonds have been languishing for three months). Nuts and seeds have delicate fats that are susceptible to heat, light, and air, so store in the refrigerator or freezer to prevent them from going rancid or sour.

Dark Leafy Greens: Look for greens that are perky and unblemished. To extend the life of your greens, wash and dry them well, then stick them in a jar of water or vase before refrigerating.

Ginger: You can use either fresh or ground ginger in smoothies. If choosing fresh, look for ginger that has smooth, thin skin and is not shriveled or wrinkled.

Green Tea and Matcha: There are many different varieties of green tea, as well as numerous brands of matcha, so experiment with the assorted types you find available. Culinary matcha is more affordable than ceremonial-grade matcha.

Oats: Rolled oats are a nice option for smoothies, though you could also choose quick-cooking oats for smoother blending (I personally enjoy the texture of thicker oats, but you might not). If gluten intolerance is an issue, purchase certified gluten-free oats. Store in the pantry.

Pomegranate: The darker the skin, the sweeter your pomegranate will be. Store in the refrigerator.

Turmeric: Purchase ground in small amounts rather than bulk for optimum freshness. Store in the pantry.

Yogurt and Kefir: Making your own yogurt and kefir is both economical and easy (see chapter 5, page 67). If you choose to purchase your yogurt or kefir instead, check labels for added sugars and preservatives; if opting for dairy, try to choose organic. Store in the refrigerator, or freeze in ice cube trays for long-term storage.

Using and Mixing Superfoods: More Is Not Always More

We have the tendency to believe that if something is good for us—diet, exercise, sleep, work—then more must automatically be better. But this usually isn't the case, especially with certain potent superfoods. Theoretically, it's possible to overdo it on any food: You'd probably feel quite ill if you ate four bunches of kale in one sitting. (And you certainly wouldn't digest and absorb the nutrients if you were eliminating that kale soon after in the bathroom!)

An advantage of many superfoods is that you don't need to use large quantities to experience the benefits. In fact, you want to avoid consuming too much. For example, turmeric is a very powerful

Saving on Superfoods

Food bills add up, so try these tips for saving on superfoods.

- **Buy in bulk where possible.** If you have the freezer space, purchasing cacao, nuts, and seeds in bulk is much more economical. Check out stores like Costco for large bags of frozen fruit, and shop your farmers' markets or grocery stores—you can often purchase ingredients at a discount if buying in large amounts. Make friends with the produce manager at your local store.
- **Purchase spices in small batches,** as you often are using these in small amounts, and unused leftovers will lose flavor, freshness, and nutritional value as they sit in your pantry unused. Check out local ethnic markets for certain spices like turmeric or for matcha, as these can potentially be cheaper there than at conventional stores.
- **Make your own nut and seed butters and nut/seed milk.** You'll save money, and at the same time, you can customize to your tastes and skip the added sugars. Make batches in bulk and freeze.
- **Look for sales,** either in person, online, or by reading sales flyers.
- **Comparison shop at different stores,** and get familiar with price points.
- **For some, online grocery shopping is more affordable** because you can shop with your list and won't be lured by promotional displays or other distractions.

spice. Adding ¼ teaspoon to your smoothie will help support your health, but blend in 2 tablespoons and your smoothie will be undrinkable.

If you're worried that a small amount won't make a difference, remember that the little pinches add up. Sure, you may not experience any change in health from a ¼-teaspoon dose of turmeric on a single day. But if you consume turmeric on a regular basis—along with making additional positive diet and lifestyle choices—you're more likely to see a shift. As I mentioned earlier, it isn't a single factor that makes or breaks our health. Dropping 1 tablespoon of turmeric into your smoothie isn't better than ¼ teaspoon, especially if you spend the rest of your day gorging on junk food. We don't need to push each superfood to its limit.

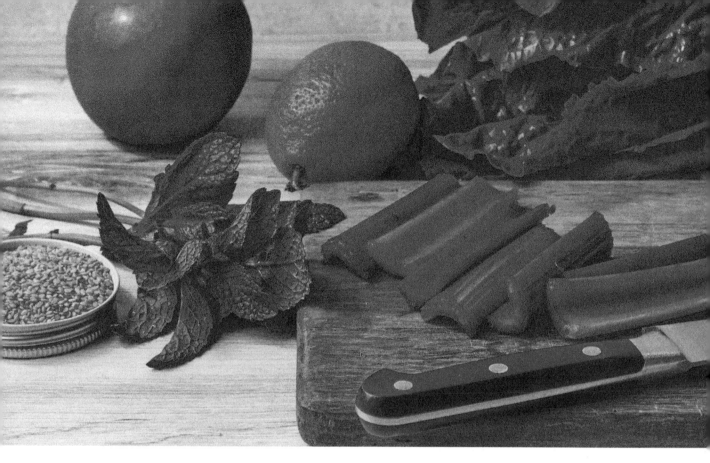

Generally, the ingredients in the second section of this book are more successful in small amounts due to their impact on overall flavor and consistency. However, some ingredients in the first section, too, can be difficult to digest if consumed in excess. To keep this all straight, the chart below offers guidelines for recommended ranges of quantities for consumption. If an ingredient is new to you—or you are new to smoothies—beginning with the minimum amount is a good idea.

Similarly, attempting to include every superfood at once will either ruin your smoothie or, at the very least, destroy the taste of any distinct ingredients at all. See the chart below for recommended combinations to boost the flavors and health benefits of your smoothies.

Note: Quantities can vary depending on your health status, activity level, and individual needs, as well as whether you intend for your smoothie to serve as a full meal replacement or a snack.

Recommended Superfood Doses (per Single Smoothie)

Superfood	Minimum Amount	Maximum Amount
Avocado	⅛ avocado	½ avocado
Bananas	¼ banana	1 whole banana
Beets, cooked, puréed	1 tablespoon	½ cup
Beets, raw, grated	2 tablespoons	¾ to 1 cup
Berries	¼ cup	1 to 1½ cups
Cacao/Cocoa	1 teaspoon	3 to 4 tablespoons
Chia Seeds	1 teaspoon	2 to 3 tablespoons
Cinnamon, ground	¼ teaspoon	2 tablespoons
Dark Leafy Greens	⅓ cup	1 to 1½ cups
Ginger, ground	⅛ teaspoon	1 to 1½ tablespoons
Ginger, raw	¼ teaspoon	1 to 2 tablespoons
Matcha	½ teaspoon	2 teaspoons
Nut/Seed Butters	1 teaspoon	2 to 3 tablespoons
Nuts/Seeds, ground	1 teaspoon	3 to 4 tablespoons
Nuts/Seeds, whole	1 teaspoon	⅓ cup
Oats	1 tablespoon	⅓ to ½ cup
Pomegranate Juice (100 percent)	2 tablespoons	1 cup
Pomegranate Seeds	1 tablespoon	¾ cup
Turmeric, ground	⅛ teaspoon	1 teaspoon
Yogurt/Kefir	1 tablespoon	¾ to 1 cup (Fermented foods can be difficult to digest at first, so work your way up. You may max out at ½ cup, so see how it goes.)

Superfood Combinations

Combination	Flavor Profile	Health Effects
Blueberries + Chocolate	Sweet/Slightly Bitter	High antioxidant value
Blueberries + Strawberries	Sweet	High antioxidant value
Chia + Yogurt	Sweet	Aids digestion, anti-inflammatory
Chocolate + Cinnamon	Sweet/Bitter	Anti-inflammatory
Cinnamon + Ginger	Sweet/Spicy	Anti-inflammatory
Greens + Avocado	Sweet/Bitter/Creamy	Fat in avocado helps vitamin and mineral absorption
Greens + Lemon	Bitter/Sour	Helps vitamin C and iron absorption
Greens + Nut/Nut Butters	Sweet/Creamy	Aids vitamin absorption, anti-inflammatory
Lemon + Green Tea	Sour/Bitter	Vitamin C in lemons helps catechin (antioxidant) absorption from green tea
Oats + Orange	Sweet	Heart healthy
Turmeric + Black Pepper	Spicy	Pepper helps absorption of turmeric constituents
Turmeric + Ginger	Spicy/Bitter	Anti-inflammatory, immunity boost
Yogurt + Banana	Tangy/Sweet	Workout recovery

Using the Recipes

The recipes in this cookbook are organized by superfood ingredient. Each chapter will feature a single superfood, with information and instructions on how to use it best, followed by recipes. Each chapter will build upon the previous ones, incorporating additional ingredients to create more flavorful, complex smoothies.

For easy reference, each recipe comes with recipe labels highlighting the primary benefits or functions of the smoothie. You can also search by recipe label in the index (see page 206).

Recipe labels include:

Anti-Aging: This smoothie contains ingredients that combat the effects of aging.

Anti-Inflammatory: This smoothie includes anti-inflammatory ingredients that can help reduce body pain.

Energy Boost: This smoothie includes ingredients that can increase energy levels.

Greens Lover: This smoothie contains green vegetables or green herbs.

Heart Healthy: This smoothie contains ingredients that benefit the cardiovascular system.

Immunity Boost: This smoothie features ingredients beneficial to the immune system.

Kid Friendly: Look for this label when you need a smoothie more pleasing to a kid's palate.

Meal Swap: This smoothie is high in protein and/or calories, so it can serve as a full meal.

Weight Loss: This smoothie contains ingredients that may aid in weight loss.

Each recipe also comes with a bonus tip:

Power Up! Tips for adding another superfood from this book for an extra health boost.

Prep Tip: Helpful food prep tips.

Simplify It! Tips to make the smoothie even easier/faster to prepare.

Substitute It! Tips for substituting ingredients to change the

What About Dairy?

Today we can choose from a wide array of dairy and nondairy options to meet our dietary needs and preferences. So how do we begin to narrow these down?

NONDAIRY

Consuming dairy-free alternatives such as nondairy milk and yogurt can have numerous benefits, ranging from improved digestion, clearer skin, and relief from sensitivities and allergies to less inflammation and better weight management.

Of course, dairy-free products may contain adverse ingredients. Watch out for added sugars or artificial sweeteners, and make sure to choose unsweetened or low-sugar plant-based milks. Nondairy products can also contain processed, low-quality oils, preservatives, and stabilizers—typically, a shorter ingredient list means a healthier, more natural product. Better yet—make your own! It only takes a few minutes to blend a Basic Nut Milk (see page 38), which you can then flavor yourself to your heart's desire.

DAIRY

If you opt to include dairy in your smoothies, I suggest you look for organic/grass-fed milk, sheep or goat milk, fermented dairy, and full-fat dairy. Here are some good reasons to choose these products:

Organic/Grass-Fed Milk. Studies comparing conventional milk with organic milk show that organic has a higher amount of anti-inflammatory omega-3 fatty acids, a higher quantity of CLA (a fat that encourages weight loss and benefits the cardiovascular system), and a lower amount of omega-6 fats, which can be inflammatory when consumed in excess.

Sheep and Goat Milk. These milks can be easier to digest than cow milk.

Fermented Dairy. Fermented products like yogurt and kefir (see chapter 5) can support healthy digestion, as some of the lactose is consumed in the fermentation process.

Full-Fat Dairy. Skip low-fat or fat-free dairy. Fat provides flavor and texture/thickness; when they remove it, companies add sugar, artificial flavors, stabilizers, and preservatives in its place.

A note on sourcing dairy: In most cases, the best dairy comes from small producers and is sold at local grocery stores. Farmers' markets are a good bet, too. However, some larger chains carry high-quality dairy from smaller local farms, so check your local supermarket.

macronutrient ratio or to address a different health effect or taste profile.

Taste Tip: Advice for improving or changing the smoothie's flavor.

Remember, you are your own best guide in the kitchen. Trust your instincts and your palate. I encourage you to use these recipes as models, not dogma. There may be times when you'd like to add more water for a thinner smoothie, or use fewer kale leaves. And if you aren't crazy about the taste of one smoothie today, tomorrow is another day!

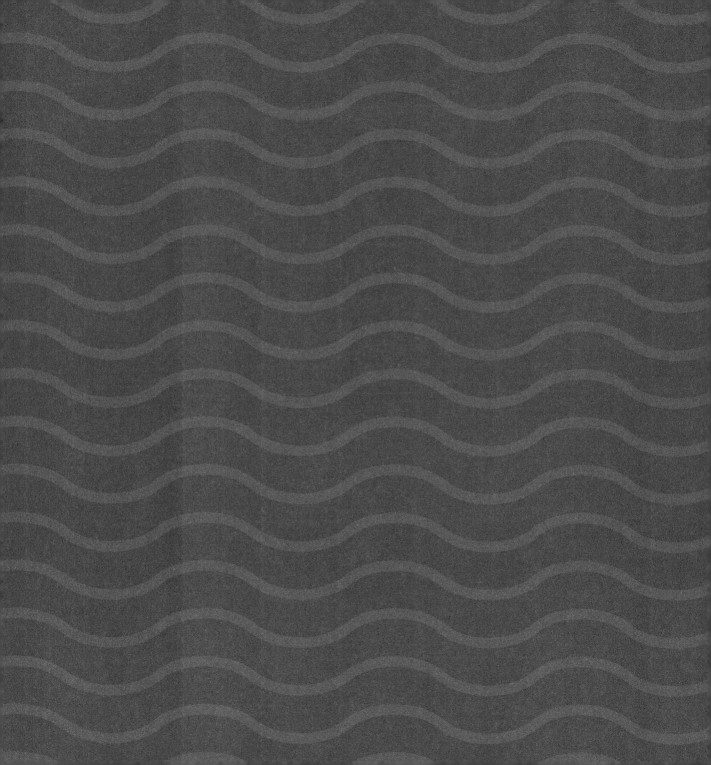

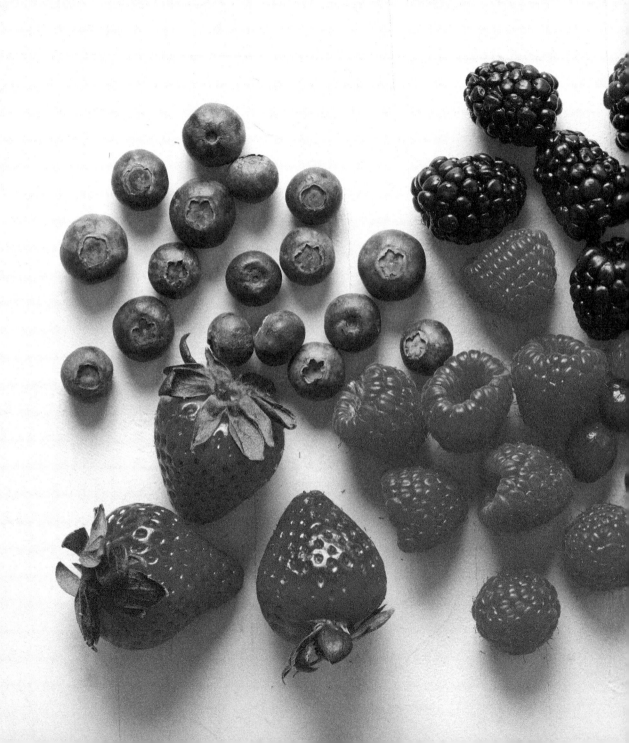

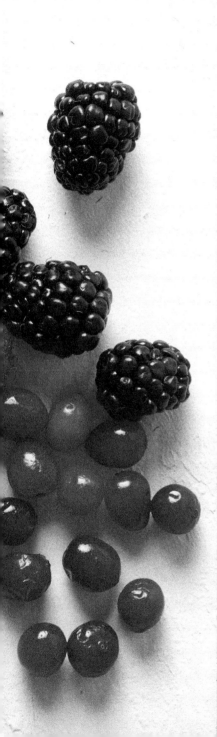

Part One

SUPERFOOD
BASE-ICS

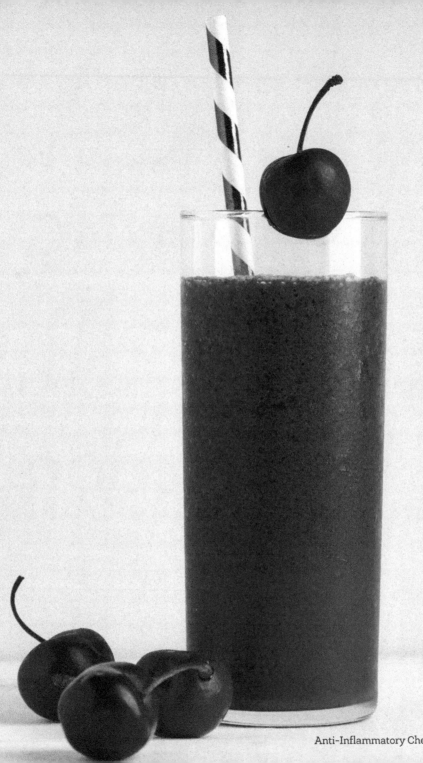

Anti-Inflammatory Cherry-Berry Smoothie, page 12

Chapter One

Common Berries

Berries aren't just a summer essential, they're staple smoothie fruits you can use to add flavor and a wallop of nutrition to your blended beverages throughout the entire year. Most notably, berries are rich in antioxidants that protect our bodies from damage. One family of berry anti-oxidant compounds called anthocyanins are responsible for their gorgeous hues. In addition, berries are packed with fiber, which benefits digestion, blood sugar balance, and cardiovascular health. Berries have been widely studied for their anti-inflammatory and anti-cancer properties, along with their ability to reduce the risk of cardiovascular, neurodegenerative, and metabolic diseases. That's a lot of power packed into one small package!

Common forms: Fresh and frozen, both of which work well in smoothies, though I prefer to use frozen to achieve a thick, frosty texture. Many berries are heavily treated with pesticides (see page 197), so I opt for organically grown when available.

Where to find them: In the produce section or freezer section of your supermarket, farmers' markets, or local farms for U-Pick. When buying fresh, remember to look for berries that are firm (rather than mushy), and check at the bottom of the container for any mold.

Prep tip: Buy berries in bulk when they are in season, and freeze to enjoy all year in smoothies. Wash, dry, and lay berries out on a parchment-lined baking sheet. Freeze until firm, then transfer to a freezer-safe container and label with the type of berry and the date. (You think you'll remember this information, but you won't!)

Blueberry-Coconut Energy Sustainer

**Anti-Inflammatory
Energy Boost**

Makes 2 (14-ounce) servings
Prep time: 5 minutes

1½ cups full-fat coconut milk
½ cup water
1½ cups frozen blueberries
¼ cup hemp seeds

Coconut milk is one of my favorite smoothie bases because it lends a luxurious texture that instantly makes your smoothie resemble a milk shake. Easy to digest, coconut milk contains antimicrobial properties, as well as healthy, anti-inflammatory fats that help us support energy levels and feel satiated. If you are concerned about the fat content, simply use equal parts coconut milk and water instead.

1. In a blender, combine the coconut milk, water, blueberries, and hemp seeds. Blend until smooth, about 1 minute, stopping the blender if needed to scrape down the sides so everything is fully incorporated.
2. Pour into two glasses and enjoy.

✳ **Power Up!** Add 1 cup of spinach for a boost of vitamins, minerals, and fiber.

PER SERVING Calories: 597; Total Fat: 49 g; Sugars: 17 g; Carbohydrates: 26 g; Fiber: 7 g; Protein: 8 g

Fragrant Strawberry-Basil Smoothie

Anti-Inflammatory
Heart Healthy
Immunity Boost

Makes 2 (12-ounce) servings
Prep time: 5 minutes

1½ cups almond milk
1½ cups frozen strawberries,
    thawed 5 to 10 minutes for
    easier blending
6 fresh basil leaves, torn in half
1 teaspoon honey or maple syrup

Basil is typically associated with savory dishes, but it makes a very aromatic and tasty addition to smoothie recipes, as well. Basil contains flavonols that are anti-inflammatory and anti-bacterial, helping us ward off infections; at the same time, it's a source of nutrients that support cardiovascular health.

1. In a blender, combine the almond milk, strawberries, basil leaves, and honey or maple syrup. Blend until smooth, about 2 minutes, stopping the blender if needed to scrape down the sides so everything is fully incorporated.
2. Pour into two glasses and enjoy.

✳ **Power Up!** Add 1 teaspoon ground cinnamon to the blender for some additional sweetness, plus extra anti-inflammatory and blood sugar–balancing benefits.

PER SERVING Calories: 113; Total Fat: 5 g; Sugars: 8 g; Carbohydrates: 15 g; Fiber: 4 g; Protein: 2 g

Raspberry-Orange Fiber Kick

Heart Healthy

Weight Loss

Makes 2 (14-ounce) servings
Prep time: 5 minutes

1 cup water (see tip)
1½ cups frozen raspberries
2 small oranges (any variety),
    peeled and cut into
    1-inch chunks
2 dates, pitted
¼ cup hemp seeds

Fiber is essential for good digestion, blood sugar balance, and satiety, and while all berries are good fiber sources, raspberries are a standout. Evidence indicates that raspberries also contain phytochemicals that help manage insulin levels and may prevent obesity by increasing metabolism and enzyme activity in our fat cells. When you combine raspberries with fiber- and antioxidant-rich oranges, you're in for a delicious, nutritious boost!

1. In a blender, combine the water, raspberries, oranges, dates, and hemp seeds. Blend until smooth, about 2 minutes, stopping the blender if needed to scrape down the sides so everything is fully incorporated.
2. Pour into two glasses and enjoy.

Substitute It! Swap half or all of the water for nondairy or dairy kefir or yogurt of your choice to provide a creamier texture, tangy flavor, and digestion-friendly probiotics.

PER SERVING Calories: 382; Total Fat: 6 g; Sugars: 55 g; Carbohydrates: 67 g; Fiber: 11 g; Protein: 5 g

Blackberry-Lime Immunity Booster

**Anti-Inflammatory
Immunity Boost**

Makes 2 (12-ounce) servings
Prep time: 5 minutes

1½ cups water
2 cups frozen blackberries
1 lime, zested, peeled, and
  quartered
2 dates, pitted

Calling all lovers of tart, acidic flavors! This combination of blackberries and lime will make your mouth pucker, but in the best way possible. As a bonus, you'll receive a high dose of vitamin C to pump up your immune system.

1. In a blender, combine the water, blackberries, lime quarters and zest, and dates. Blend until smooth, about 2 minutes, stopping the blender if needed to scrape down the sides so everything is fully incorporated.
2. Pour into two glasses and enjoy.

✳ **Power Up!** Add a few mint leaves for their digestive benefits and flavor.

PER SERVING Calories: 95; Total Fat: 1 g; Sugars: 13 g; Carbohydrates: 24 g; Fiber: 9 g; Protein: 2 g

Sweet 'n' Tart Cranberry Smoothie

Anti-Inflammatory
Heart Healthy

Makes 2 (14-ounce) servings
Prep time: 5 minutes

1½ cups water or nondairy or
   dairy milk of choice
1 cup frozen strawberries, thawed
   5 to 10 minutes for easier
   blending
⅔ cup fresh or frozen cranberries
¼ cup unsweetened
   shredded coconut
2 teaspoons maple syrup or honey

Most of us aren't used to eating cranberries whole and unadorned. We either consume them dried and sweetened or during the holiday season in sugar-laden cranberry sauce. Whole cranberries, though rather tart, add a delicious flavor profile to smoothies, as well as a bump of antioxidants that benefit the cardiovascular system. Sweet strawberries are the perfect foil for cranberries, seamlessly offsetting their natural sour taste.

1. In a blender, combine the water, strawberries, cranberries, coconut, and maple syrup. Blend until smooth, about 2 minutes, stopping the blender if needed to scrape down the sides so everything is fully incorporated.
2. Taste, and add more maple syrup if it's too tart.
3. Pour into two glasses and enjoy.

Taste Tip: Channel the holiday season by adding fresh grated ginger and ground nutmeg, cinnamon, allspice, and cloves.

PER SERVING Calories: 144; Total Fat: 8 g; Sugars: 10 g; Carbohydrates: 16 g; Fiber: 5 g; Protein: 1 g

Raspberry Lemonade Fountain of Youth

Anti-Aging
Weight Loss

Makes 2 (12-ounce) servings
Prep time: 5 minutes

1½ cups water or nondairy or
    dairy milk of choice
1½ cups frozen raspberries
Zest and juice of 1 lemon (see tip)
1 (4-inch) piece of cucumber, cut
    into 1-inch chunks
2 dates

When we add spoonfuls of sugar to traditional lemonade, we aren't just masking the fruit flavor. High glycemic index, sugary foods break down the collagen and elastin in our skin, leading to skin aging and sagging. Thankfully raspberries, lemon, and cucumber are all rich in vitamin C, which supports collagen production and keeps us as youthful as we are in our memories.

1. In a blender, combine the water, raspberries, lemon zest and juice, cucumber, and dates. Blend until smooth, about 2 minutes, stopping the blender if needed to scrape down the sides so everything is fully incorporated.
2. Pour into two glasses and enjoy.

Prep Tip: Zest and juice lemons in large batches, then freeze in ice cube trays for easy use in smoothies and other recipes.

PER SERVING Calories: 233; Total Fat: 1 g; Sugars: 48 g; Carbohydrates: 59 g; Fiber: 9 g; Protein: 2 g

Tropical Mango-Strawberry Crowd Pleaser

Energy Boost

Kid Friendly

Makes 2 (14-ounce) servings
Prep time: 5 minutes

1½ cups water or nondairy or
    dairy milk of choice
½ cup full-fat coconut milk
1 cup frozen strawberries,
    thawed 5 to 10 minutes for
    easier blending
1 cup frozen mango

Most berries are naturally sweet on their own, but adding tropical fruits like mango, pineapple, or papaya can make berry smoothies more appealing to young palates. The sweetness also has the potential to hide other superfoods and veggies like dark leafy greens, chia seeds, zucchini, or cucumber!

1. In a blender, combine the water, coconut milk, strawberries, and mango. Blend until smooth, about 2 minutes, stopping the blender if needed to scrape down the sides so everything is fully incorporated.
2. Pour into two glasses and enjoy.

✶ **Power Up!** Add in freshly grated ginger or cinnamon for its anti-inflammatory properties.

PER SERVING Calories: 212; Total Fat: 15 g; Sugars: 18 g;
Carbohydrates: 22 g; Fiber: 4 g; Protein: 2 g

Anti-Inflammatory Cherry-Berry Smoothie

Anti-Inflammatory
Heart Healthy

Makes 2 (14-ounce) servings
Prep time: 5 minutes

1½ cups water or nondairy or
    dairy milk of choice
1 cup frozen, pitted cherries
½ cup frozen raspberries (see tip)
½ cup frozen blueberries (see tip)
2 tablespoons almond butter

Grab an extra dose of antioxidants and anti-inflammatory nutrients by including cherries in your smoothie recipe. Their compounds have been known to aid with inflammatory conditions such as heart disease and arthritis and can even help you sleep and lift your mood. Sweet cherries are the way to go here, and unless you love getting sprayed with cherry juice, opt for frozen, pitted ones.

1. In a blender, combine the water, cherries, raspberries, blueberries, and almond butter. Blend until smooth, about 2 minutes, stopping the blender if needed to scrape down the sides so everything is fully incorporated.
2. Pour into two glasses and enjoy.

Substitute It! Substitute any berries in this recipe: Use just one variety or a mix of several, adding up to 1 cup.

PER SERVING Calories: 235; Total Fat: 9 g; Sugars: 29 g; Carbohydrates: 40 g; Fiber: 7 g; Protein: 5 g

Peppery Cardamom-Berry Smoothie

Anti-Inflammatory

Weight Loss

Makes 2 (14-ounce) servings
Prep time: 5 minutes

1½ cups water or nondairy or
  dairy milk of choice
1 cup frozen blueberries
1 cup frozen blackberries
1 teaspoon vanilla extract
⅛ teaspoon ground cardamom
  (see tip)

Cardamom is a warm, peppery spice that has been studied for its anti-inflammatory and anti-cancer properties, as well as for its potential to reduce some cardiovascular risk, oxidative stress, and insulin sensitivity—all of which can lead to obesity. A little goes a long way with cardamom, so just don't add too much!

1. In a blender, combine the water, blueberries, blackberries, vanilla, and cardamom. Blend until smooth, about 2 minutes, stopping the blender if needed to scrape down the sides so everything is fully incorporated.
2. Pour into two glasses and enjoy.

Substitute It! If you are unable to locate ground cardamom, try 1 teaspoon fresh ginger or 1 teaspoon ground cinnamon.

PER SERVING Calories: 79; Total Fat: 1 g; Sugars: 11 g; Carbohydrates: 18 g; Fiber: 6 g; Protein: 2 g

Sweet Roasted Berry Smoothie

Energy Boost
Kid Friendly

Makes 3 (8-ounce) servings
Prep time: 5 minutes
Cook time: 30 minutes

2 cups mixed fresh berries of
  choice (if using strawberries,
  halve them; see tip)
1 tablespoon coconut sugar
  (optional—depends on
  whether you are using very
  tart berries, like cranberries
  or blackberries)
¾ cup water
¾ cup full-fat coconut milk
¼ cup hemp seeds
Handful ice cubes or crushed ice
  (optional)

Most fresh berries in season will be sweet and juicy, but you can intensify their sweetness and flavor by roasting them for a special treat. Your kitchen will smell heavenly while you bake your berries—you'll have to stop yourself from swiping them while they cool to have at least a few left for your smoothie!

1. Preheat the oven to 350°F. Line a baking sheet with parchment paper for less cleanup, or use a glass or ceramic dish for roasting.
2. Spread the berries out on the parchment paper or dish. Sprinkle with coconut sugar (if using).
3. Roast for 20 to 30 minutes, until the berries have softened considerably and released a lot of their juices. Cool completely before using in your smoothie. The larger the berries, the more time they will need to roast.
4. In a blender, combine the berries and their juices with the water, coconut milk, hemp seeds, and ice (if using). Blend until smooth, about 1 minute, stopping the blender if needed to scrape down the sides so everything is fully incorporated.
5. Pour into three glasses and enjoy.

Prep Tip: Double or triple the quantity of mixed berries to have extra on hand to spoon over oatmeal, granola, yogurt, ice cream, pancakes, waffles, or parfaits, or for snacking. You can also freeze roasted berries for use in future smoothies.

PER SERVING Calories: 290; Total Fat: 20 g; Sugars: 7 g; Carbohydrates: 11 g; Fiber: 3 g; Protein: 5 g

Forever Young Apple-Berry Smoothie

Anti-Aging

Heart Healthy

Makes 2 (12-ounce) servings
Prep time: 5 minutes

1 cup water or nondairy or dairy
milk of choice
2 apples, cored and cut into
2-inch pieces (see tip)
½ cup frozen raspberries
½ cup frozen strawberries,
thawed 5 to 10 minutes for
easier blending

The well-worn phrase "An apple a day keeps the doctor away" persists for a reason! Apples are packed with fiber, vitamins, and minerals, and are noted for their anti-inflammatory, anti-cancer, anti-obesity, and anti-diabetic effects. Thousands of apple varieties are grown around the world, so choose whichever you have available. Sweeter varieties like Gala, Fuji, Honeycrisp, Ambrosia, Red and Golden Delicious, Pink Lady, and Jonagold are some of my favorites.

1. In a blender, combine the water, apples, raspberries, and strawberries. Blend until smooth, about 2 minutes, stopping the blender if needed to scrape down the sides so everything is fully incorporated.
2. Pour into two glasses and enjoy.

Prep Tip: The apple skin contains several nutrients, plus fiber, so don't peel it!

PER SERVING Calories: 144; Total Fat: 1 g; Sugars: 27 g; Carbohydrates: 38 g; Fiber: 8 g; Protein: 1 g

Anything Goes Berry Smoothie

**Anti-Inflammatory
Immunity Boost**

Makes 2 (14-ounce) servings
Prep time: 5 minutes

1½ cups water or nondairy or
   dairy milk of choice
2½ cups frozen or fresh berries
   of choice
2 dates
3 tablespoons almond butter

This is a handy recipe to call on when you've got berries in the refrigerator losing their firmness. Or you discover an old, freezer-burned bag of berries, all stuck together. All are welcome in the blender!

1. In a blender, combine the water, berries, dates, and almond butter. Blend until smooth, about 2 minutes, stopping the blender if needed to scrape down the sides so everything is fully incorporated.
2. Pour into two glasses and enjoy.

✳ **Power Up!** While you're cleaning out the refrigerator, toss in a few handfuls of dark leafy greens or wilted herbs for extra nutrition.

PER SERVING Calories: 270; Total Fat: 14 g; Sugars: 19 g; Carbohydrates: 32 g; Fiber: 9 g; Protein: 7 g

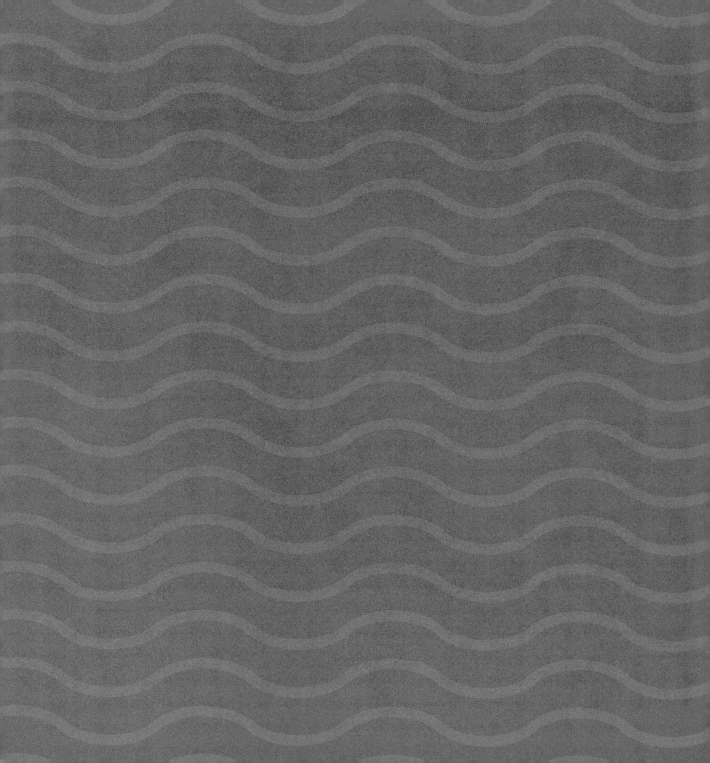

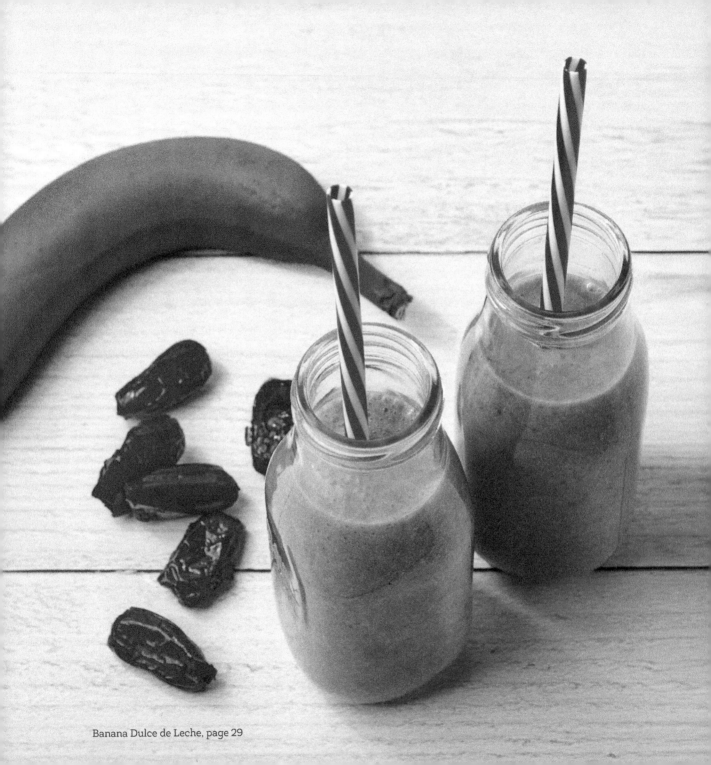

Banana Dulce de Leche, page 29

Chapter Two

Bananas

Considering their sweet flavor and creamy texture, it's no surprise that bananas are one of the world's most highly consumed fruits. But bananas aren't just winning popularity contests: There's a lot of substance behind their attractive exterior!

Bananas are well-known as a great source of potassium, an electrolyte mineral that can help lower blood pressure, maintain healthy heart function, and aid with muscle recovery after exercise. They also contain a range of B vitamins that support energy levels as well as the nervous system and are a good source of fiber.

There are some differences between eating unripe bananas (the green/yellow ones) and ripe bananas. Unripe bananas are starchier, firmer, and less sweet, but they contain a form of carbohydrate called "resistant starch" that acts as a prebiotic, which feeds the good bacteria in the colon. Once bananas ripen, becoming spotted and dark, those starches turn into sugar, making them sweeter and easier to digest.

In smoothies I prefer using very ripe bananas for their sweetness and easy digestibility, letting them ripen until they are practically covered in brown spots before freezing. Because of their sweetness, however, I use them in small amounts: about half a banana per smoothie. Depending on your health goals, you can adjust the sweetness of your smoothie, using unripe, semi-ripe, or fully ripe bananas.

Common forms: There are several different banana varieties, but what you'll typically find in most grocery stores is the long and yellow Cavendish bananas. Plantains, another member of the banana family, are increasing in popularity and are starchier than Cavendish bananas. They are usually consumed cooked rather than raw and are often treated more like a potato than a banana, which is why I don't recommend them in these smoothie recipes.

Where to find them: In the produce section. Remember to talk to your produce manager, as some grocery stores will set aside brown bananas for customers who bake or make smoothies. They may even give you a good deal on them; plus, buying brown bananas saves you the time you'd have to wait for yellow bananas to ripen at home.

Prep tip: If your bananas are not ripe, place them in a paper bag and close the top. To speed the process, you can also add an apple to the bag. Once they ripen (with plenty of large, brown spots), line a large baking sheet with parchment paper. Peel the bananas, slice into 1-inch pieces, then freeze on the prepared baking sheet for a couple of hours (to prevent the slices from sticking together). Transfer the slices to a freezer-safe container, and they are ready to blend in your smoothies. About 4 to 5 slices is equal to half a banana; 8 to 10 is equivalent to a whole.

Banana-Kale Green Smoothie

Greens Lover

Immunity Boost

Makes 2 (8-ounce) servings

Prep time: 5 minutes

1 cup water or nondairy or dairy
milk of choice

1 large leaf curly kale, torn into
pieces (about 1 cup)

1 frozen banana

1 orange, peeled and chopped into
1-inch chunks (see tip)

¼ cup hemp seeds

If you are struggling with including strongly flavored greens in your smoothie, adding sweet fruits such as bananas is the answer. Here they alleviate some of the bitterness of kale, but if you find the kale still too harsh for your taste, try a milder green such as spinach or romaine instead.

1. In a blender, combine the water, kale, banana, orange, and hemp seeds. Blend until smooth, about 2 minutes, stopping the blender if needed to scrape down the sides so everything is fully incorporated.

2. Pour into two glasses and enjoy.

Prep Tip: For a thicker texture, freeze your orange chunks for an hour before preparing this smoothie.

PER SERVING Calories: 232; Total Fat: 5 g; Sugars: 16 g; Carbohydrates: 28 g; Fiber: 4 g; Protein: 6 g

Banana Pumpkin Pie Smoothie

Immunity Boost

Makes 2 (8-ounce) servings
Prep time: 5 minutes

1 cup full-fat coconut milk
1 cup pumpkin purée (homemade
  or canned)
1 frozen banana
1 tablespoon maple syrup
⅛ teaspoon ground nutmeg
Pinch salt

Winter squashes such as pumpkin offer a broad range of nutrients to support us during the harsh winter months. Their wealth of vitamins A and C keep our immune systems strong, while their fiber content helps balance blood sugar levels. With its blend of fall flavors like pumpkin, nutmeg, and maple, this smoothie tastes like drinking pie—you can't go wrong with that!

1. In a blender, combine the coconut milk, pumpkin purée, banana, maple syrup, nutmeg, and salt. Blend until smooth, about 1 minute, stopping the blender if needed to scrape down the sides so everything is fully incorporated.
2. Pour into two glasses and enjoy.

⁎ **Power Up!** For anti-inflammatory boosts, add 1 teaspoon ground cinnamon and ½ teaspoon ground ginger. These will also help replicate even further that traditional pumpkin pie flavor!

PER SERVING Calories: 397; Total Fat: 29 g; Sugars: 21 g; Carbohydrates: 37 g; Fiber: 8 g; Protein: 5 g

Banana-Raspberry Fiber Fuel

Energy Boost
Greens Lover
Weight Loss

Makes 2 (8-ounce) servings
Prep time: 5 minutes

1¼ cups water or nondairy or
    dairy milk of choice
½ cup fresh spinach
2 tablespoons ground flaxseed
    (see tip)
1 cup frozen raspberries
1 frozen banana

Between the spinach, flax, and fruit, this smoothie has fiber firing on all cylinders! I love fiber because it keeps your digestive system humming, supports cardiovascular health, helps you maintain a healthy weight, and balances blood sugar. If you're not accustomed to consuming fruits and veggies regularly, try adding an extra ¼ to ⅓ cup liquid to avoid bloating or constipation.

1. In a blender, combine the water, spinach, flaxseed, raspberries, and banana. Blend until smooth, about 2 minutes, stopping the blender if needed to scrape down the sides so everything is fully incorporated.
2. Pour into two glasses and enjoy.

Substitute It! Flax is rich in anti-inflammatory omega-3s, has a gelling, mucilaginous quality, and absorbs liquid easily. So does chia! If you prefer, you can easily swap ground chia for ground flax in this recipe.

PER SERVING Calories: 243; Total Fat: 5 g; Sugars: 35 g; Carbohydrates: 51 g; Fiber: 11 g; Protein: 5 g

Strawberry-Banana Omega-3 Booster

Immunity Boost

Kid Friendly

Makes 2 (10-ounce) servings
Prep time: 5 minutes

1¼ cups water or nondairy or
   dairy milk of choice
1½ cups frozen strawberries,
   thawed 5 to 10 minutes for
   easier blending
1 frozen banana
2 fresh mint leaves (optional)
¼ cup hemp seeds

You won't have problems convincing children to eat fruit with this sweet smoothie that contains near the recommended daily amount of vitamin C. Hemp seeds, rich in anti-inflammatory and brain-supportive omega-3s, are a secret weapon here, because you won't be able to taste them. If you can't find hemp seeds, swap for another nut or seed your family enjoys.

1. In a blender, combine the water, strawberries, banana, mint leaves (if using), and hemp seeds. Blend until smooth, about 2 minutes, stopping the blender if needed to scrape down the sides so everything is fully incorporated.
2. Pour into two glasses and enjoy.

☀ **Power Up!** Add ¼ cup plain, unsweetened nondairy or dairy yogurt or kefir of your choice (store-bought or homemade, page 70) to the blender for digestion-friendly probiotics, extra fat, and tanginess.

PER SERVING Calories: 190; Total Fat: 5 g; Sugars: 14 g; Carbohydrates: 23 g; Fiber: 4 g; Protein: 4 g

Almond Butter and Banana Pick-Me-Up

Energy Boost
Kid Friendly

Makes 2 (6-ounce) servings
Prep time: 5 minutes

1 cup nondairy or dairy milk
   of choice
½ cup water
1 frozen banana
¼ cup almond butter

This smoothie allows the banana to shine and is incredibly easy to pull together at a moment's notice. It's an ideal after-school or post-activity snack because it supplies you with nutrients for recovery but won't stuff you to the gills so that you or your little ones have no appetite for the next meal.

1. In a blender, combine the milk, water, banana, and almond butter. Blend until smooth, about 1 minute, stopping the blender if needed to scrape down the sides so everything is fully incorporated.
2. Pour into two glasses and enjoy.

✳ **Power Up!** Add a tablespoon of cacao for a chocolate kick, or for a more substantial protein boost, opt for a scoop of your favorite protein powder.

PER SERVING Calories: 265; Total Fat: 19 g; Sugars: 9 g; Carbohydrates: 23 g; Fiber: 7 g; Protein: 11 g

Blueberry-Banana Slimmer

Anti-Inflammatory

Heart Healthy

Weight Loss

Makes 2 (8-ounce) servings

Prep time: 5 minutes

---

1 cup water or nondairy or dairy milk of choice

1½ cups frozen blueberries

1 frozen banana

¼ cup pecans (see tip)

1 tablespoon freshly squeezed lemon juice

Blueberries and bananas make a fantastic flavor combination in baking. Who doesn't love blueberry-banana bread, muffins, or cookies? Experience this joy in a glass by blending this blueberry-banana smoothie, which also happens to support weight loss and heart health as a side bonus.

1. In a blender, combine the water, blueberries, banana, pecans, and lemon juice. Blend until smooth, about 1 minute, stopping the blender if needed to scrape down the sides so everything is fully incorporated.
2. Pour into two glasses and enjoy.

Substitute It! Substitute the pecans with any other nut or seed you have on hand, or skip them entirely.

PER SERVING Calories: 222; Total Fat: 12 g; Sugars: 19 g; Carbohydrates: 31 g; Fiber: 6 g; Protein: 3 g

Banana, Mango, and Orange Vitamin C Lift

Anti-Aging
Immunity Boost
Kid Friendly

Makes 2 (8-ounce) servings
Prep time: 5 minutes

¼ cup cashews, soaked for
    2 hours in cold water and
    drained (see tip)
1 cup water or nondairy or dairy
    milk of choice
1 cup frozen mango
1 frozen banana
1 large orange, juiced

Feeling blue? Brighten up your day with this bright and sunny smoothie filled with vitamin C. It not only helps bolster your immune system but also keeps your skin supple and strong.

1. In a blender, combine the cashews, water, mango, banana, and orange juice. Blend until smooth, about 2 minutes, stopping the blender if needed to scrape down the sides so everything is fully incorporated.
2. Pour into two glasses and enjoy.

Simplify It! No cashews on hand? Try 2 tablespoons cashew butter instead.

PER SERVING Calories: 247; Total Fat: 7 g; Sugars: 27 g; Carbohydrates: 41 g; Fiber: 6 g; Protein: 5 g

Banana Dulce de Leche

Kid Friendly

Makes 2 (6-ounce) servings
Prep time: 5 minutes

For the date paste

1 cup dates, pitted
1 cup warm water

For the smoothie

1 cup full-fat coconut milk
1 frozen banana
¼ cup date paste, or more to taste
½ teaspoon vanilla extract
Pinch salt

This smoothie/milk shake is delicious on its own, but if you're in a decadent mood, try adding a scoop of your favorite (nondairy or dairy of your choice) vanilla ice cream. Yep, I went there.

To make the date paste

1. In a medium bowl, soak the dates in water for 10 minutes, or longer if your dates are very firm.
2. Combine the dates and water in a blender or food processor, and blend together until a thick paste forms. For a thinner consistency, continue to blend water into the paste, adding 1 tablespoon of water at a time.
3. Store in the refrigerator. The paste lasts for about a week. If you won't be using it right away, stick it in the freezer. Leftover paste can be used as a sweetener in baking, to make more smoothies, or in oatmeal.

To make the smoothie

1. In a blender, combine the coconut milk, banana, date paste, vanilla, and salt. Blend until smooth, about 2 minutes, stopping the blender if needed to scrape down the sides so everything is fully incorporated.
2. Pour into two glasses and enjoy.

✴ **Power Up!** To amp up the protein content, add several tablespoons of nut butter or a scoop of your favorite protein powder.

PER SERVING Calories: 394; Total Fat: 29 g; Sugars: 26 g; Carbohydrates: 37 g; Fiber: 6 g; Protein: 4 g

Banana, Grapefruit, and Apple Antioxidant Smoothie

Anti-Aging

Immunity Boost

Makes 2 (10-ounce) servings

Prep time: 5 minutes

---

1 cup full-fat coconut milk

½ cup water

1 small pink or red grapefruit, peeled and cut into 1-inch chunks (see tip)

1 frozen banana

2 apples, chopped into 1-inch chunks

¼ cup hemp seeds

Grapefruit, with its bitter-tart flavor, can be the toughest to love out of all the citrus fruits. But there's good reason to acquire a taste for it: Pink and red grapefruit contain a significant quantity of lycopene, an antioxidant that helps fight cancerous tumors and promotes heart health. The banana and apple in this recipe, as well as the fat from the coconut milk, help cut the bitterness.

1. In a blender, combine the coconut milk, water, grapefruit, banana, apples, and hemp seeds. Blend until smooth, about 1 minute, stopping the blender if needed to scrape down the sides so everything is fully incorporated.
2. Pour into two glasses and enjoy.

Taste Tip: Still too tart? Juice the grapefruit over a fine mesh strainer, and use the liquid rather than the whole fruit.

PER SERVING Calories: 586; Total Fat: 34 g; Sugars: 39 g; Carbohydrates: 56 g; Fiber: 10 g; Protein: 7 g

Banana Bread Green Energy Spike

Anti-Aging

Energy Boost

Greens Lover

Makes 2 (6-ounce) servings

Prep time: 5 minutes

1 cup water

½ cup walnuts

1 cup spinach

1 frozen banana

2 dates or 2 tablespoons date paste (see Banana Dulce de Leche, page 29)

1 teaspoon vanilla extract

⅛ teaspoon ground allspice

⅛ teaspoon ground nutmeg

Pinch salt

This smoothie recipe combines the flavor notes of your favorite banana bread with the nutritional boost of dark leafy greens. The unstrained walnut milk prepared at the beginning of the recipe adds texture and fiber to the smoothie without being too gritty. However, if you prefer a silkier feel, simply strain the walnut milk before proceeding with the rest of the recipe.

1. In a blender, combine the water and walnuts and blend until smooth. Stop the blender and add the spinach, banana, dates, vanilla, allspice, nutmeg, and salt. Blend until smooth, about 2 minutes, stopping the blender if needed to scrape down the sides so everything is fully incorporated.
2. Pour into two glasses and enjoy.

Taste Tip: Add a teaspoon of cinnamon to enhance the flavor, and if you're feeling adventurous, some ground ginger and turmeric as well.

PER SERVING Calories: 299; Total Fat: 22 g; Sugars: 14 g; Carbohydrates: 25 g; Fiber: 5 g; Protein: 6 g

Coffee-Banana Perk-Up

Energy Boost

Makes 2 (8-ounce) servings
Prep time: 5 minutes

1 cup full-fat coconut milk
1 cup chilled coffee or coffee alternative
1 frozen banana
¼ cup hemp seeds

Add a twist to your morning coffee with the addition of banana and coconut milk for luxurious creamy sweetness. If you're not a coffee fan—or are attempting to cut back—try exploring herbal coffee alternatives that use dandelion root and chicory, which have a similar, but milder, coffee flavor.

1. In a blender, combine the coconut milk, coffee, banana, and hemp seeds. Blend until smooth, about 1 minute, stopping the blender if needed to scrape down the sides so everything is fully incorporated.
2. Pour into two glasses and enjoy.

✳ **Power Up!** Convert your smoothie from coffee to mocha by adding 1 tablespoon of cacao powder.

PER SERVING Calories: 459; Total Fat: 34 g; Sugars: 11 g; Carbohydrates: 20 g; Fiber: 4 g; Protein: 6 g

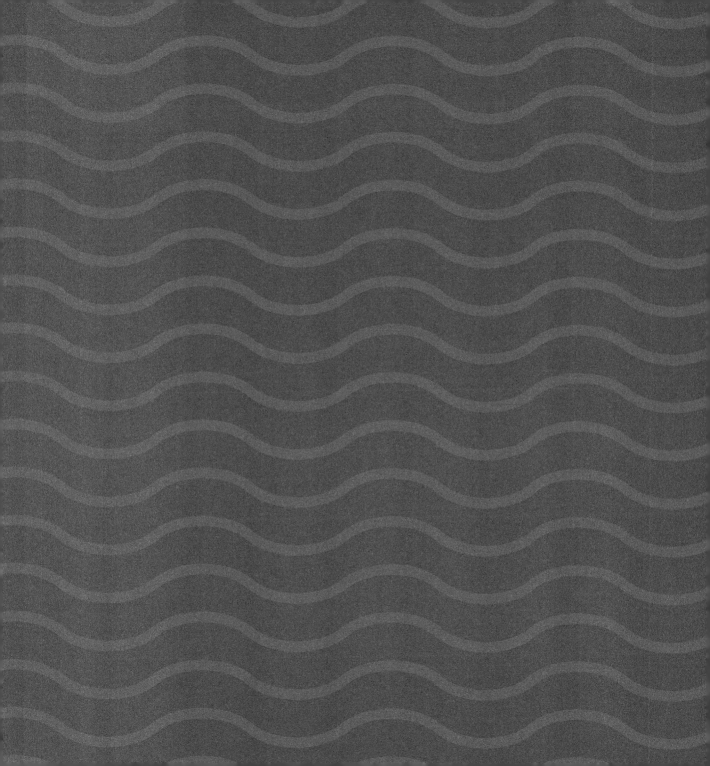

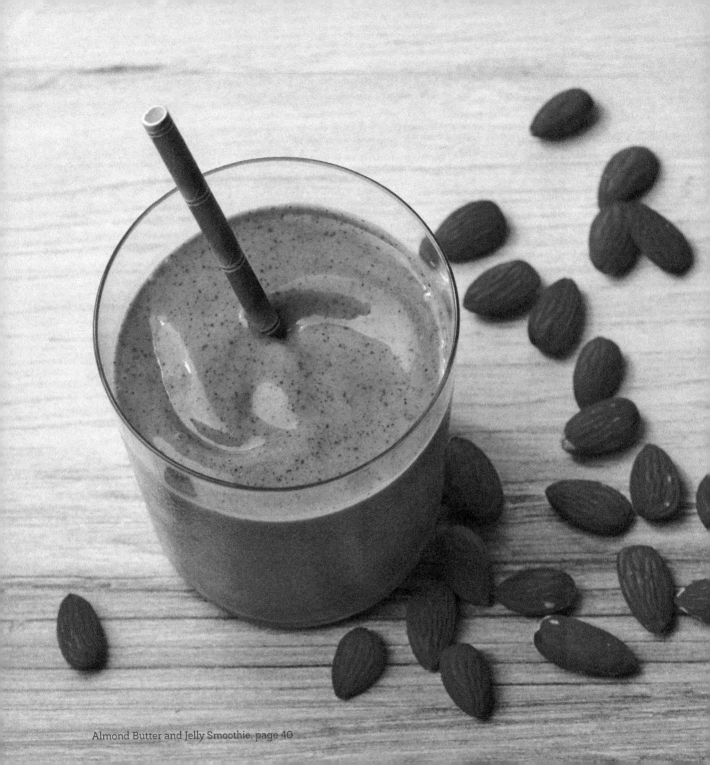

Almond Butter and Jelly Smoothie, page 40

Chapter Three

Common Nuts and Seeds

I'm going to restrain myself from using any nut-related puns here, as nuts and seeds are serious business! Ranging from the teeny tiny to approximately the size of one's thumbnail, the minute dimensions of common nuts and seeds belie their enormous nutritional value. And with so many varieties to choose from, nuts can easily keep your smoothies exciting while giving them serious staying power.

Nuts and seeds are rich sources of protein, fat, vitamins, minerals, and antioxidants. There is a wide body of research on how they help us: Nut and seed consumption improves cholesterol levels; balances blood sugar; promotes weight loss and prevents weight gain; boosts the immune system and modulates inflammation; bolsters memory, mood, and cognition; encourages the growth of good bacteria in the gut; and lowers the risk of heart disease, type 2 diabetes, and cancer. Whew!

Some of the nuts and seeds used in this chapter include sesame seeds, flaxseed, pumpkin seeds, sunflower seeds, cashews, almonds, pecans, walnuts, and hazelnuts. This is not an exhaustive list, and you are welcome to swap in different nuts or seeds you enjoy or that are easily available to you.

Common forms: You can find nuts whole, chopped/slivered, and ground as well as in the form of nut/seed butters and milks.

Where to find them: Purchase nuts in the bulk section or in packages at the grocery store. Nut milks and nut butters should be in the middle aisles, or you may even find them fresh at local farmers' markets. You only want the freshest nuts, so if you are buying from bulk bins, remember to purchase from stores with a high turnover. If you are purchasing store-bought nut milks, look for brands that are low in sugar or have no sugar. They will all have preservatives to keep them shelf stable. Choose nuts or butters that only contain nuts/seeds, rather than additional sugar or oils.

Prep tip: Because they contain delicate fats, nuts and seeds are vulnerable to heat, light, and air. Keep them fresh by storing in the refrigerator or freezer.

I prefer buying whole, raw, and unsalted nuts (usually in bulk). That way, I can flavor, roast, or spice them as I choose. Nuts that have already been roasted, salted, or processed (chopped/slivered) are usually more expensive, and you can't control what temperatures they were exposed to or what was added to them.

Pulverize nuts to a meal or powder to make your own instant protein powder. When grinding, do so in smaller batches (one or two cups at a time, or two if you are making a lot of smoothies for others in your household), and store in a sealed jar in the refrigerator. Grinding nuts and seeds exposes them to more heat, light, and air, which can damage their nutrients and encourage quicker rancidity.

Soaking nuts and seeds can help them blend more quickly; soak for 2 to 6 hours (small seeds will require less time than larger nuts like almonds). The soaking process also makes nuts and seeds easier to digest, as it removes some antinutrients that interfere with digestion.

Batch-blend nut milks and store them in the freezer in jars and ice cube trays to use in a variety of recipes. Don't forget to label them!

The recipes here use soaked nuts and seeds, whole nuts and seeds, ground nuts and seeds, nut and seed milks, and nut butters. Depending on the strength of your blender, you may want to blend whole or soaked nuts or seeds with liquids before adding the remaining ingredients. For even easier blending, you can always opt for using nut or seed butters in your smoothies instead.

Note: The recipes in this cookbook are peanut-free. Technically, peanuts are not a nut, they're a legume, and a very common allergen. They can also contain high levels of aflatoxins, a family of toxins that can compromise the liver and suppress healthy immune function, and are carcinogenic.

Basic Nut Milk

. . . .

Heart Healthy

Weight Loss

Makes 2 to 4 cups
Prep time: 5 minutes

---

1 cup nuts or seeds (or a mix of both), soaked for 2 to 6 hours
2 to 4 cups water
Pinch salt
Sweetener of choice (optional)

Nut or seed milks offer flavor and creaminess to smoothies and are simple to make at home, allowing you to ditch sugars and preservatives. If separation occurs (as there are no additives here), just give the milk a quick shake. Then flavor and sweeten as desired—adding chocolate is always a tasty option!

1. Drain and rinse your nuts and seeds. In a blender, combine the water, nuts and seeds, salt, and sweetener (if using). Two cups of water will yield a thick milk; the more water you add, the thinner it will become. Blend until smooth and creamy, about 2 minutes, stopping the blender if needed to scrape down the sides so everything is fully incorporated.

2. If using a fine mesh strainer: Place over a large bowl, then pour the milk through it. Press down on the nut pulp with the back of a spoon to squeeze all the milk out.

3. If using a nut milk bag: Place the bag in a large bowl, and pour the milk through it. Squeeze the milk out, leaving the pulp.

4. Store in a sealed jar or container in the refrigerator, and freeze in jars (leaving an inch of headspace at the top) or ice cube trays. The nut milk will last, refrigerated, for about 4 days.

Prep Tip: Don't forget to save your nut milk pulp for use in baking, or dry it out and use it as breadcrumbs.

PER SERVING (1 CUP) Calories: 40; Total Fat: 3 g; Sugars: 0 g; Carbohydrates: 0 g; Fiber: 0 g; Protein: 1 g

Basic Nut Butter

Energy Boost
Kid Friendly
Weight Loss

Makes about 2 cups
Prep time: 15 minutes
Cook time: 10 minutes, plus at least
30 minutes to cool

---

3 cups nuts or seeds of choice
Pinch salt (optional)

Taste Tip: Superfood boosts that appear later in this book, including cinnamon, cacao, ginger, turmeric, and matcha, all make lovely flavor additions to homemade nut butters. For a natural sweetness, try maple syrup or honey. You can even make a swirled version with two flavors. Hello, chocolate-swirled almond butter!

Ever notice how everything contains sugar these days? Even a simple food like nut butter is no longer safe, topped up with sugar and often unhealthy oils, too. Creating fresh nut or seed butter requires a little bit of time and patience, yet it's not labor intensive—and the results are worth it. Any nut or seed works in this recipe, or you can even mix a bunch together. If you have a large food processor container, you'll probably want to double this recipe!

1. Preheat the oven to 350°F.
2. Spread the nuts out in an even layer on a large baking sheet. Bake for 7 to 10 minutes, until lightly golden and fragrant. Smaller seeds will take less time, while larger nuts may take longer. Keep a close eye on them. Remember that they will continue to cook as they cool.
3. Remove from the oven and allow to cool for at least half an hour.
4. In a food processor, blend the nuts or seeds, stopping and scraping down the sides as necessary. This may take 10 to 15 minutes.
5. Add the salt (if using), and blend once more.
6. Pour the nut or seed butter into a jar. If the butter has warmed while blending, allow it to cool before sealing the lid, and store in the refrigerator. The butter should last, refrigerated, for at least 4 to 6 weeks.

PER SERVING (1 TABLESPOON) Calories: 67; Total Fat: 6 g; Sugars: 0 g; Carbohydrates: 3 g; Fiber: 1 g; Protein: 3 g

Almond Butter and Jelly Smoothie

Kid Friendly

Makes 2 (8-ounce) servings
Prep time: 5 minutes

1 cup almond milk
1 cup frozen strawberries, thawed
   5 to 10 minutes for easier
   blending
1 frozen banana
¼ cup almond butter, plus extra
   for drizzling
Chocolate chips, for serving
   (optional)

The lunchbox classic is reinvented without the bread or peanut butter—and it tastes so darn good you won't miss either. If almond butter isn't your bag, try any nut or seed butter you prefer instead!

1. In a blender, combine the almond milk, strawberries, banana, and almond butter. Blend until smooth, about 2 minutes, stopping the blender if needed to scrape down the sides so everything is fully incorporated.
2. Pour into two glasses and enjoy. Drizzle with extra almond butter, or sprinkle with chocolate chips (if using) for an extra treat.

Simplify It! No strawberries? Add your favorite frozen berries, or ¼ cup preprepared jam.

PER SERVING Calories: 309; Total Fat: 20 g; Sugars: 14 g; Carbohydrates: 28 g; Fiber: 7 g; Protein: 9 g

Lemony-Cashew Vitamin C Burst

Anti-Inflammatory

Immunity Boost

Makes 2 (9-ounce) servings
Prep time: 5 minutes

2 cups cashew milk
2 small lemons, zested, peeled, seeded, and cut into chunks
1 frozen banana
3 tablespoons cashew butter
2 dates, pitted
1 teaspoon vanilla extract
Pinch salt
Handful of ice (optional)

We often use lemon zest or lemon juice and don't consider using the whole lemon. Yes, it's a sour fruit, but combining it with some sweeter ingredients makes this smoothie taste like a lemon pie or tart. And you're getting an influx of immune-boosting vitamin C!

1. In a blender, combine the cashew milk, lemon zest and chunks, banana, cashew butter, dates, vanilla, salt, and ice (if using). Blend until smooth, about 2 minutes, stopping the blender if needed to scrape down the sides so everything is fully incorporated.
2. Pour into two glasses and enjoy.

Simplify It! No time to make cashew milk? Double the amount of cashew butter and use 2 cups water, which will create a cheater's cashew milk when everything is blended together.

PER SERVING Calories: 265; Total Fat: 14 g; Sugars: 14 g; Carbohydrates: 33 g; Fiber: 4 g; Protein: 6 g

Cashew-Caramel Mineral Fuel

Anti-Aging

Energy Boost

Kid Friendly

Makes 2 (8-ounce) servings

Prep time: 5 minutes

1 cup cashew milk

½ cup full-fat coconut milk

½ cup cashews, soaked for at least 2 hours, then drained

1 frozen banana

¼ cup date paste (see Banana Dulce de Leche, page 29) or 2 dates, pitted

Handful of ice (optional)

Cashews are one of my favorite nuts to use in smoothies because they are neutral and pair well with many flavors. They're also rich in magnesium—great for relaxation and bone health—as well as copper, a mineral that bolsters anti-oxidant production to aid our bones, skin, hair, and energy levels. There's more to this smoothie than meets the eye!

1. In a blender, combine the cashew milk, coconut milk, cashews, banana, date paste, and ice (if using). Blend until smooth, about 2 minutes, stopping the blender if needed to scrape down the sides so everything is fully incorporated.

2. Pour into two glasses and enjoy.

Substitute It! If nut allergies are an issue, this smoothie works well with tahini. Simply omit the cashew milk and cashews, use 1½ cups coconut milk (or a mix of nondairy or dairy milk of your choice and water), and add ⅓ cup tahini. This will also make a smoothie higher in calcium.

PER SERVING Calories: 389; Total Fat: 28 g; Sugars: 15 g; Carbohydrates: 32 g; Fiber: 5 g; Protein: 7 g

Multi-Textured Almond-Raspberry Smoothie

Energy Boost

Greens Lover

Heart Healthy

Meal Swap

Weight Loss

Makes 2 (8-ounce) servings
Prep time: 5 minutes

1½ cups water
¾ cup spinach, lightly packed
1 cup frozen raspberries
¼ cup ground almonds or
   almond meal
10 whole almonds, chopped

Almonds are rich in monounsaturated fats, also found in olive oil, which is heavily used in Mediterranean diets. These fats help support good cardiovascular health, but also balance blood sugar levels and encourage weight loss. The mix of almond textures in this smoothie—ground and chopped—adds interest and encourages you to "chew" your smoothie for better digestion.

1. In a blender, combine the water, spinach, raspberries, and ground almonds. Blend until smooth, about 2 minutes, stopping the blender if needed to scrape down the sides so everything is fully incorporated.
2. Pour into two glasses, sprinkle the chopped almonds on top, and enjoy.

⁎ **Power Up!** For more almond power and flavor, use almond milk instead of water.

PER SERVING Calories: 245; Total Fat: 10 g; Sugars: 27 g; Carbohydrates: 37 g; Fiber: 8 g; Protein: 5 g

Pumpkin Seed–Peachy Keen Vitality Kick

Heart Healthy
Immunity Boost

Makes 2 (12-ounce) servings
Prep time: 5 minutes

1½ cups water or nondairy or
   dairy milk of choice
1½ cups frozen peaches
½ cup frozen mango
¼ cup pumpkin seed butter

Pumpkin seeds are a highly nutritious addition to any smoothie: They contain a wealth of minerals, including zinc for healthy immune function and reproductive wellness, manganese for blood sugar balance and strong bones, and copper. If you are cooking with pumpkin, don't toss the seeds—toast them in the oven for making pumpkin seed butter or milk, or just for munching on as a handy snack (see Prep Tip).

1. In a blender, combine the water, peaches, mango, and pumpkin seed butter. Blend until smooth, about 2 minutes, stopping the blender if needed to scrape down the sides so everything is fully incorporated.
2. Pour into two glasses and enjoy.

Prep Tip: To toast pumpkin seeds, preheat the oven to 350°F. Spread them on a baking sheet in an even layer and bake for 10 to 20 minutes, until lightly golden brown. Stir halfway through toasting time to ensure even browning, and check frequently near the end to avoid burning.

✴ **Power Up!** Mild leafy greens are an excellent and nutritious addition here, providing extra minerals to help with nutrient absorption. Try a handful of spinach or romaine, which won't change the flavor.

PER SERVING Calories: 262; Total Fat: 18 g; Sugars: 14 g; Carbohydrates: 20 g; Fiber: 4 g; Protein: 7 g

Sunny Sunbutter Surprise

Anti-Inflammatory

Greens Lover

Heart Healthy

Meal Swap

Makes 2 (12-ounce) servings
Prep time: 5 minutes

1½ cups water or nondairy or
    dairy milk of choice
1 cup spinach, lightly packed
1 cup frozen mango
1 cup frozen pineapple
¼ cup sunflower seed butter
1 tablespoon freshly squeezed
    lemon juice

Of all the seed butters, sunflower seed butter—especially when roasted—tastes the most like peanut butter to me. It's great paired with chocolate, berries, or tropical fruits, and nutritionally, it's a good source of vitamin E, which helps prevent cardiovascular diseases—plus, it contains a trace amount of the mineral selenium that inhibits cancer cells. This bright and sweet smoothie is a lovely way to start the day!

1. In a blender, combine the water, spinach, mango, pineapple, sunflower seed butter, and lemon juice. Blend until smooth, about 2 minutes, stopping the blender if needed to scrape down the sides so everything is fully incorporated.
2. Pour into two glasses and enjoy.

✳ **Power Up!** A teaspoon of fresh ginger adds some extra zing, as well as anti-inflammatory benefits.

PER SERVING Calories: 281; Total Fat: 16 g; Sugars: 20 g; Carbohydrates: 33 g; Fiber: 3 g; Protein: 8 g

"Naked" Hazelnut-Honey Smoothie

Heart Healthy

Meal Swap

Makes 2 (8-ounce) servings
Prep time: 5 minutes

1¼ cups water
½ cup toasted hazelnuts (see
    Prep Tip)
1 frozen banana
2 tablespoons raw honey
2 tablespoons flaxseed

Hazelnuts are a versatile nut often paired with chocolate or coffee. These combinations are delicious, of course, but they overshadow the nut's true flavor. While you can certainly add some cacao or chilled coffee here, this recipe, featuring its "naked" form, allows the beautiful hazelnut flavor to shine.

1. In a blender, combine the water, hazelnuts, banana, honey, and flaxseed. Blend until smooth, about 1 minute, stopping the blender if needed to scrape down the sides so everything is fully incorporated.
2. Pour into two glasses and enjoy.

Simplify It! If you aren't able to toast the hazelnuts ahead of time, just skip this step and proceed with the recipe.

Prep Tip: To toast hazelnuts, preheat the oven to 350°F. Spread the nuts on a baking sheet in an even layer, and bake for 10 to 15 minutes, until lightly golden brown. Stir halfway through toasting time to ensure even browning, and check frequently near the end to avoid burning.

PER SERVING Calories: 287; Total Fat: 15 g; Sugars: 25 g; Carbohydrates: 37 g; Fiber: 6 g; Protein: 6 g

Heart-Healthy Halvah Smoothie

. . . .

Anti-Inflammatory

Energy Boost

Heart Healthy

Makes 2 (8-ounce) servings

Prep time: 5 minutes

¾ cup nondairy or dairy milk
  of choice

¾ cup water

1 frozen banana

¼ cup tahini (raw or roasted)

2 tablespoons raw honey

1 date, pitted

1 teaspoon vanilla extract

Pinch salt

Halvah is a dense Middle Eastern treat made with sesame paste (tahini) and sugar. Sesame seeds are small but mighty. They are rich in a variety of minerals, particularly calcium to support bone health and muscle/nerve function, as well as a sesamin, a special plant fiber that helps lower cholesterol. To make this recipe vegan, use maple syrup instead of honey.

1. In a blender, combine the milk, water, banana, tahini, honey, date, vanilla, and salt. Blend until smooth, about 1 minute, stopping the blender if needed to scrape down the sides so everything is fully incorporated.
2. Pour into two glasses and enjoy.

Taste Tip: Tahini from unhulled sesame seeds is slightly more nutritious than from hulled, but it will also have a more bitter flavor. I prefer to use hulled sesame seeds: They hold most of the health benefits of sesame, but are more palatable in smoothies and other recipes.

PER SERVING Calories: 344; Total Fat: 19 g; Sugars: 28 g; Carbohydrates: 41 g; Fiber: 6 g; Protein: 7 g

Sweet Cherry-Pecan Delight

Heart Healthy
Immunity Boost
Meal Swap
Weight Loss

Makes 2 (12-ounce) servings
Prep time: 5 minutes

½ cup pecans
1½ cups water or nondairy or
    dairy milk of choice
1½ cups frozen cherries
½ cup frozen cauliflower florets
1 frozen banana

Love the sweetness of pecans? You're in luck. A study in the journal *Nutrients* examined the blood work of participants who ate a handful of pecans daily for a month and found that pecans reduced their risk of cardiovascular disease and Type 2 diabetes. While frozen cauliflower might seem like an odd ingredient for a smoothie, it adds creaminess, fiber, and vitamin C, and when blended with fruit, you won't even notice it.

1. In a blender, combine the pecans and water. Blend for 30 seconds. Add the cherries, cauliflower, and banana, and blend until smooth, about 2 minutes, stopping the blender if needed to scrape down the sides so everything is fully incorporated.
2. Pour into two glasses and enjoy.

✳ **Power Up!** Add 1 teaspoon of ground cinnamon for an anti-inflammatory boost, or ½ cup of yogurt for flavor and probiotic benefits. Or add them both!

PER SERVING Calories: 297; Total Fat: 20 g; Sugars: 19 g; Carbohydrates: 31 g; Fiber: 7 g; Protein: 5 g

Pecan-Walnut Carrot Cake Smoothie

Anti-Inflammatory

Heart Healthy

Immunity Boost

Meal Swap

Makes 2 (14-ounce) servings

Prep time: 5 minutes

---

3 tablespoons pecans

3 tablespoons walnuts

1½ cups water

¾ cup full-fat coconut milk

1¼ cups grated carrots
(about 1 large)

1 cup frozen pineapple chunks

Pinch ground nutmeg

Pinch ground allspice

Pinch salt

Chopped walnuts, pecans, or
shredded coconut, for topping
(optional)

Yellow and orange veggies like carrots are rich in beta-carotene, a plant pigment our bodies convert into vitamin A for wound healing, and that supports our immune systems, vision, and cardiovascular health. If you have any cooked carrots on hand, you can use those instead of raw, if you'd like—your smoothie may taste a bit sweeter, but there's nothing wrong with that!

1. In a blender, combine the pecans and walnuts with the water and coconut milk. Blend for 30 seconds. Add the carrots, pineapple, nutmeg, allspice, and salt. Blend until smooth, about 2 minutes, stopping the blender if needed to scrape down the sides so everything is fully incorporated.
2. Pour into two glasses, top with chopped nuts or shredded coconut (if using), and enjoy!

✳ **Power Up!** Add ¼ cup of rolled oats to this smoothie for extra B vitamins and fiber, as well as some additional thickness and texture. This smoothie also works well as a smoothie bowl.

PER SERVING Calories: 393; Total Fat: 34 g; Sugars: 14 g; Carbohydrates: 23 g; Fiber: 6 g; Protein: 5 g

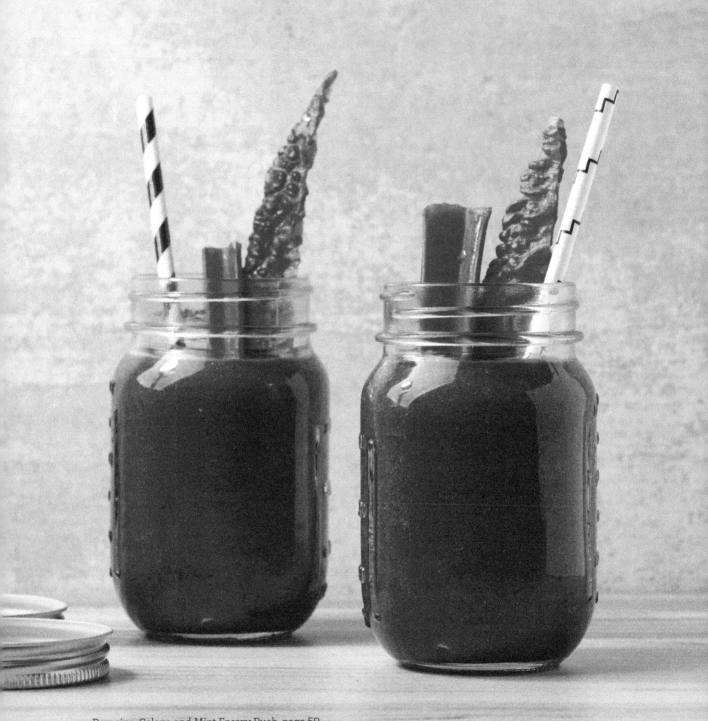

Romaine, Celery, and Mint Energy Rush, page 59

Chapter Four

Dark Leafy Greens

Dark leafy greens contain such a comprehensive spectrum of nutrients, I don't even know where to begin! Nevertheless, I need to start somewhere, so first let's discuss what makes them bright green: the pigment chlorophyll, also known as the "blood" of plants. Chlorophyll has antioxidant, anti-inflammatory, and anti-cancer properties, and along with minerals like iron found in greens, helps support red blood cell production.

Greens contain an array of B vitamins known for boosting energy levels and balancing the nervous system, as well as fiber for digestive support. They also contain the antioxidant vitamins A, C, and E that protect our cells from damage and boost immunity, plus vitamin K, magnesium, and calcium for bone health. They even possess small amounts of protein and healthy fats (omega-3s). In short, dark leafy greens are multitalented and truly hustle to keep you healthy.

Since they are nutrient-rich, many dark leafy greens can be strong and bitter in taste. Spinach is a great starter for green smoothies because it is mild and neutral—it will change the color of your smoothie, but you won't really taste it. Baby greens are also a lovely option because they are gentler on the palate than their mature counterparts.

As you become accustomed to consuming dark leafy greens, begin to experiment with stronger varieties like kale, chard, collards, arugula, watercress, dandelion, or whatever greens grow in your area. Start off with small amounts of stronger greens, and cut them with milder greens like spinach and lettuces (for example, try ½ cup spinach plus ½ cup kale, or ¾ cup spinach plus ¼ cup watercress), and see how it goes.

Greens are an incredibly easy way to add more nutrition to your smoothies. Once you begin experimenting, you may find it tough to go back to smoothies without them!

Common forms: You can find dark leafy greens in bunches, bundles, or loose-leaf in clamshells or plastic bags. (The latter is usually pre-washed, too.)

Where to find them: Search for dark leafy greens in the produce and freezer sections of your supermarket, or at local farmers' markets. I personally prefer to purchase unpackaged greens as often as possible. While washed, bagged greens are convenient, the packaging contributes to environmental waste. If you are buying packaged greens, try to purchase brands that come in packages that are recyclable or biodegradable (and be sure to recycle them properly).

Prep tip: To extend the life of your greens, remember to wash and dry them well, and place them in a jar filled with water (like flowers in a vase). Wrap the exposed greens with a bag or tea towel to create a "biodome" effect before refrigerating. When using greens that have thick stems, like kale, collards, and chards, save the stems for juicing, or chop them for stir-fries.

Don't forget that you can save the greens from the tops of vegetables like beets, turnips, and carrots to use in smoothies, pestos, sauces, and more—though to decrease their bitterness, you may want to blanch them first, before throwing them into your blender.

Spinach, Raspberry, and Banana Starter Smoothie

Greens Lover

Kid Friendly

Makes 2 (10-ounce) servings

Prep time: 5 minutes

1½ cups water or nondairy or
   dairy milk of choice
1 cup spinach, tightly packed
1 cup frozen raspberries
1 frozen banana
1 date, pitted

This is a fantastic introduction for those who are new to or hesitant about green smoothies. All you will taste are the sweet raspberries and banana, while the spinach, with all its nutritional power casually—and quietly—hangs out in the background.

1. In a blender, combine the water, spinach, raspberries, banana, and date. Blend until smooth, about 2 minutes, stopping the blender if needed to scrape down the sides so everything is fully incorporated.
2. Pour into two glasses and enjoy.

Substitute It! Feeling brave? Swap the spinach for kale once you are ready to take on stronger dark leafy greens.

PER SERVING Calories: 100; Total Fat: 1 g; Sugars: 13 g; Carbohydrates: 25 g; Fiber: 6 g; Protein: 2 g

Mango-Pineapple Tropical Green Smoothie

Anti-Inflammatory

Greens Lover

Immunity Boost

Kid Friendly

Meal Swap

Makes 2 (14-ounce) servings
Prep time: 5 minutes

1½ cups full-fat coconut milk
   (see tip)
½ cup water
1 cup spinach, tightly packed
1 cup frozen mango
1 cup frozen pineapple
1 frozen banana
¼ cup hemp seeds

Bright green and sweet, this tropical smoothie is stuffed to the brim with antioxidants, particularly vitamin C, which helps reduce inflammation and boost immunity. Creamy coconut milk fuses it all together with an extra tropical punch. Just close your eyes, pretend you're on a beach, and listen for the rolling waves!

1. In a blender, combine the coconut milk, water, spinach, mango, pineapple, banana, and hemp seeds. Blend until smooth, about 2 minutes, stopping the blender if needed to scrape down the sides so everything is fully incorporated.
2. Pour into two glasses and enjoy.

Simplify It! If you're short on time or don't have coconut milk in the pantry, use water instead.

PER SERVING Calories: 680; Total Fat: 49 g; Sugars: 33 g; Carbohydrates: 47 g; Fiber: 8 g; Protein: 9 g

Blueberry-Herb Explosion

Greens Lover

Immunity Boost

Makes 2 (14-ounce) servings
Prep time: 5 minutes

1½ cups water or nondairy or
    dairy milk of choice
1 cup spinach, tightly packed
¾ cup fresh parsley, lightly
    packed (including stems)
4 fresh mint sprigs, stemmed
1 cup frozen blueberries
¼ cup almond butter

When building smoothies, don't forget to include herbs!
Green herbs are immensely powerful, and you don't need
to use much to receive their benefits. Some herbs are more
well-suited to smoothies than others: Fresh parsley, cilantro,
mint, basil, and even small amounts of rosemary and sage
can all work well. Parsley is an outstanding source of antioxidants like vitamins K and C, while mint aids digestion and
prevents harmful bacterial growth.

1. In a blender, combine the water, spinach, parsley, mint,
   blueberries, and almond butter. Blend until smooth, about
   2 minutes, stopping the blender if needed to scrape down
   the sides so everything is fully incorporated.
2. Pour into two glasses and enjoy.

Substitute It! Some of us adore cilantro, while others think it
tastes like soap (it's not your fault if you hate it—it's genetic).
If you're a cilantro lover, for a twist, try swapping it for
the parsley.

PER SERVING Calories: 256; Total Fat: 19 g; Sugars: 9 g;
Carbohydrates: 19 g; Fiber: 4 g; Protein: 7 g

Kale-Apple Nutrient Powerhouse

Anti-Aging

Anti-Inflammatory

Greens Lover

Makes 2 (10-ounce) servings
Prep time: 5 minutes

1½ cups water or nondairy or
    dairy milk of choice
2 curly kale leaves, torn
    into pieces
½ cup spinach
1 apple, any variety, cored and cut
    into 1-inch chunks
1 frozen banana
1 date, pitted

Kale has exploded in popularity in recent years: The number of farms growing kale more than doubled between 2007 and 2012, while production rose by 60 percent in the same time period. Kale is the darling of soups, smoothies, and chips for a reason: It's highly dense in nutrients, including antioxidants that prevent inflammation, encourage detoxification, and reduce cancer risk. Though kale can be bitter, the sweetness of the apple, banana, and date helps counter it.

1. In a blender, combine the water, kale, spinach, apple, banana, and date. Blend until smooth, about 2 minutes, stopping the blender if needed to scrape down the sides so everything is fully incorporated.
2. Pour into two glasses and enjoy.

Taste Tip: If this smoothie is still too green and strong, throw in another half cup of sweet fruit.

PER SERVING Calories: 157; Total Fat: 0 g; Sugars: 22 g; Carbohydrates: 39 g; Fiber: 6 g; Protein: 3 g

Hidden Zucchini Green Smoothie

Anti-Inflammatory

Greens Lover

Makes 2 (10-ounce) servings
Prep time: 5 minutes

1½ cups water or nondairy or
   dairy milk of choice
¾ cup chopped zucchini, fresh
   or frozen
¾ cup spinach, tightly packed
1 cup frozen mango
2 tablespoons flaxseed

Move over, zucchini noodles. There's a new way to enjoy zucchini: With its mild flavor, zucchini makes a welcome addition to smoothies. From a nutritional standpoint, zucchini is a good idea, too, as it contains a broad spectrum of minerals. It's widely available in the summertime, but if you can't find it, any summer squash will do.

1. In a blender, combine the water, zucchini, spinach, mango, and flaxseed. Blend until smooth, about 2 minutes, stopping the blender if needed to scrape down the sides so everything is fully incorporated.
2. Pour into two glasses and enjoy.

✶ **Power Up!** Add ½ cup of yogurt or kefir for extra creaminess and digestive benefits.

PER SERVING Calories: 130; Total Fat: 5 g; Sugars: 12 g; Carbohydrates: 19 g; Fiber: 6 g; Protein: 5 g

Romaine, Celery, and Mint Energy Rush

Energy Boost

Greens Lover

Makes 2 (14-ounce) servings
Prep time: 5 minutes

1½ cup water or nondairy or dairy
  milk of choice

½ head romaine lettuce, chopped
  (about 2½ to 3 cups)

3 celery stalks, chopped into
  1-inch chunks

4 fresh mint sprigs, stemmed

1 cup frozen pineapple

1 green apple, cored and cut into
  1-inch chunks

¼ cup hemp seeds or
  sesame seeds

1 tablespoon freshly squeezed
  lemon juice

Here is a zesty, slightly sweet smoothie, giving lettuce and celery a starring role. These ingredients are sometimes overshadowed by a zippy salad dressing or meatier fixings in a stew, but they are more than just the low-calorie, bland vegetables we might think—lettuce and celery are great sources of fiber and antioxidants, too.

1. In a blender, combine the water, romaine, and celery. Blend until finely chopped, about 1 minute—it doesn't need to be completely smooth at this point.
2. Add the mint, pineapple, apple, hemp seeds, and lemon juice, and blend until smooth, about 2 minutes, stopping the blender if needed to scrape down the sides so everything is fully incorporated.
3. Pour into two glasses and enjoy.

✳ **Power Up!** Add half an avocado for a creamier texture and more healthy fats.

PER SERVING Calories: 236; Total Fat: 6 g; Sugars: 21 g; Carbohydrates: 30 g; Fiber: 5 g; Protein: 4 g

Chard and Berry Detox Smoothie

Anti-Inflammatory

Greens Lover

Weight Loss

Makes 2 (14-ounce) servings
Prep time: 5 minutes

1½ cups water or nondairy or dairy milk of choice

4 or 5 Swiss chard leaves, stemmed, leaves torn into pieces (see tip)

2 cups mixed berries

1 frozen banana

1 date

¼ cup sunflower seed butter

All dark leafy greens are special in their own way, but with multicolored stems, Swiss chard is one of the prettiest. Those vibrant colors—a rainbow of white, pale green, yellow, orange, pink, and red—come from compounds called betalains, which help enhance our detoxification processes and reduce damage and inflammation in the body.

1. In a blender, combine the water, chard, berries, banana, date, and sunflower seed butter. Blend until smooth, about 2 minutes, stopping the blender if needed to scrape down the sides so everything is fully incorporated.
2. Pour into two glasses and enjoy.

Prep Tip: Save your chard stems to sauté for your next stir-fry, soup, or stew. If you're not using them right away, simply freeze them for later.

PER SERVING Calories: 352; Total Fat: 16 g; Sugars: 21 g; Carbohydrates: 47 g; Fiber: 9 g; Protein: 10 g

Strawberry-Spinach Building Block Smoothie

Anti-Aging

Greens Lover

Immunity Boost

Kid Friendly

Makes 2 (14-ounce) servings
Prep time: 5 minutes

1½ cups water or nondairy or
   dairy milk of choice
1½ cups spinach, lightly packed
2 cups frozen strawberries,
   thawed 5 to 10 minutes for
   easier blending
1 orange, peeled and chopped into
   1-inch chunks
¼ cup almond butter

There's something about strawberries that makes the "medicine" of dark leafy greens so much easier to swallow when they are combined. This simple smoothie is quick to prepare and acts like a blank canvas that can be dressed up with a variety of the superfoods introduced later in this book.

1. In a blender, combine the water, spinach, strawberries, orange, and almond butter. Blend until smooth, about 2 minutes, stopping the blender if needed to scrape down the sides so everything is fully incorporated.
2. Pour into two glasses and enjoy.

✳ **Power Up!** Toss in ⅓ cup pomegranate arils for an antioxidant and immunity boost.

PER SERVING Calories: 301; Total Fat: 19 g; Sugars: 19 g; Carbohydrates: 31 g; Fiber: 7 g; Protein: 6 g

Glowing Skin Green Smoothie

Anti-Aging

Anti-Inflammatory

Greens Lover

Meal Swap

Makes 2 (14-ounce) servings
Prep time: 5 minutes

1½ cups water
½ cup unsweetened or freshly
   squeezed orange juice
1 cup spinach, lightly packed
½ cup walnuts
1 cup frozen mango
1 papaya, cut into 1-inch chunks
½ cup raspberries (see tip)
½ cup frozen cherries (see tip)
2 tablespoons ground flaxseed

We all know that beauty stems from within, and I'm not just talking about a sparkling personality. A bright, youthful glow is supported by a host of nutrients: Vitamin C for collagen synthesis keeps our skin firm, antioxidants like vitamins A and C protect us from the harmful effects of the sun, and omega-3 fatty acids reduce inflammation associated with skin conditions like dermatitis, acne, and eczema, while hydration maintains suppleness. This smoothie holds all of these essential nutrients in spades!

1. In a blender, combine the water, orange juice, spinach, walnuts, mango, papaya, raspberries, cherries, and flax-seed. Blend until smooth, about 2 minutes, stopping the blender if needed to scrape down the sides so everything is fully incorporated.
2. Pour into two glasses and enjoy.

Substitute It! If you don't have raspberries or cherries on hand, any berry will do.

PER SERVING Calories: 455; Total Fat: 28 g; Sugars: 34 g; Carbohydrates: 52 g; Fiber: 13 g; Protein: 11 g

Kiwi-Chard Vitamin C Booster

Greens Lover

Immunity Boost

Meal Swap

Makes 2 (10-ounce) servings

Prep time: 5 minutes

1½ cups water or nondairy or
 dairy milk of choice

4 Swiss chard leaves, stemmed,
 leaves torn into pieces (see tip)

3 kiwis, quartered

1 frozen banana

⅓ cup cashews, soaked for
 2 hours and drained, or ¼ cup
 cashew butter

Bright green kiwis are an outstanding source—even better than the orange—of the antioxidant vitamin C, which helps bolster our immune systems, protect our skin from damage, and enhance our absorption of iron. The kiwi's fuzzy, brownish-green skin stores much of the fruit's vitamin C and fiber for blood sugar balance and digestion. It's edible, so be sure not to peel it when adding to your smoothie!

1. In a blender, combine the water, chard, kiwis, banana, and cashews. Blend until smooth, about 2 minutes, stopping the blender if needed to scrape down the sides so everything is fully incorporated.
2. Pour into two glasses and enjoy.

Substitute It! Any leafy green can replace the chard: Spinach, baby kale, or romaine all work well, or mix a few greens together.

PER SERVING Calories: 260; Total Fat: 10 g; Sugars: 19 g; Carbohydrates: 40 g; Fiber: 7 g; Protein: 7 g

Peppery Green Smoothie

Anti-Inflammatory

Greens Lover

Heart Healthy

Makes 2 (8-ounce) servings
Prep time: 5 minutes

1½ cups water or nondairy or
    dairy milk of choice
½ cup arugula, lightly packed
½ cup watercress, lightly packed
½ cup spinach, lightly packed
1 pear, cut into 1-inch chunks
1 frozen banana
1 tablespoon freshly squeezed
    lemon juice

Compounds in arugula and watercress, both members of the brassica family (the same group with other veggie members like broccoli, cauliflower, kale, bok choy, Brussels sprouts, and cabbage), have been studied for their anti-cancer and health-supportive properties. These benefits come with a spicy, peppery taste some may find hard to handle. But if you can develop the taste for them, blending these greens in your smoothie adds an impressive kick of both flavor and nourishment.

1. In a blender, combine the water, arugula, watercress, spinach, pear, banana, and lemon juice. Blend until smooth, about 2 minutes, stopping the blender if needed to scrape down the sides so everything is fully incorporated.

2. Pour into two glasses and enjoy.

Substitute It! Too spicy? Swap either the arugula or watercress for more spinach.

PER SERVING Calories: 99; Total Fat: 1 g; Sugars: 14 g; Carbohydrates: 25 g; Fiber: 4 g; Protein: 2 g

Green Chamomile-Cherry Soother

Anti-Inflammatory

Greens Lover

Heart Healthy

Immunity Boost

Makes 2 (14-ounce) servings
Prep time: 5 minutes

1½ cups chilled chamomile tea (see tip)
1 cup spinach, lightly packed
1 cup frozen, pitted cherries
¾ cup frozen strawberries, thawed 5 to 10 minutes for easier blending
¼ cup almond butter

Chamomile has been used for thousands of years as a therapeutic herb, but only recently have we discovered the details of how and why it is so beneficial. Among its many qualities and uses, chamomile combats anxiety and trouble sleeping, stimulates the immune system, and reduces inflammation. It may also reduce the risk of cardiovascular disease, and it has antimicrobial and antibacterial properties, which suit it to topical wound healing. I feel more relaxed just talking about it!

1. In a blender, combine the chamomile, spinach, cherries, strawberries, and almond butter. Blend until smooth, about 2 minutes, stopping the blender if needed to scrape down the sides so everything is fully incorporated.
2. Pour into two glasses and enjoy.

Prep Tip: Brew a large batch of chamomile tea and freeze the extra in freezer-safe containers or ice cube trays for future smoothies.

PER SERVING Calories: 275; Total Fat: 19 g; Sugars: 16 g; Carbohydrates: 27 g; Fiber: 5 g; Protein: 6 g

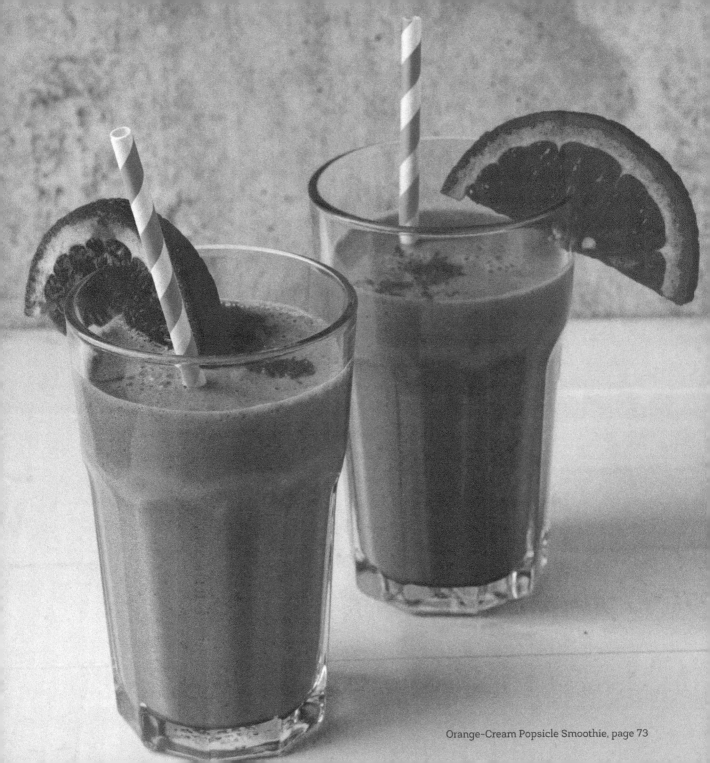

Orange-Cream Popsicle Smoothie, page 73

Chapter Five

Yogurt and Kefir

Yogurt and kefir are fermented dairy products that add protein, fat, and probiotics to smoothie recipes. They are tangy, sour, and delicious, yet with all the selections that line the dairy case, how do you know which to choose?

Kefir is thin (it's intended to be consumed as a beverage), is fermented at room temperature using kefir grains, has more fat and protein than yogurt, and contains a different range of cultures.

Yogurt, on the other hand, is thick and can be devoured with a spoon. It's fermented with heat using a variety of cultures that produce diverse flavors, thicknesses, and textures.

You may have heard that products like yogurt and kefir are excellent sources of probiotics, which can help cultivate beneficial bacteria in your gut, leading to better overall digestive health. This is true! Yet probiotics have a much greater impact on health beyond the walls of the intestines. Since around 70 to 80 percent of our immune system lives within the gut, probiotics help support the immune system. Many neurotransmitters also originate in the digestive tract, meaning good digestive health also benefits the brain.

Research on kefir indicates that it has cholesterol-lowering properties, along with antibacterial and antimicrobial activities; it also accelerates wound healing, suppresses tumors, can ease allergies and asthma, and improves digestion. Yogurt has demonstrated similar digestive benefits and it aids weight maintenance and lowers the risk of diabetes. Some research indicates that combining yogurt with fruit enhances the nutritional properties of both: This is true food synergy!

I am personally lactose intolerant, and have not consumed dairy products for more than a decade. Instead, I choose dairy-free yogurt and kefir alternatives. If you are able to consume dairy, the fermentation process helps gobble up some of the lactose and makes the nutrients more available for your body to use. Dairy products sourced from sheep and goat milk can be easier to digest than cow dairy.

Common forms: Kefir and yogurt made from dairy sources including cow, sheep, and goat milk are all available, as are vegan alternatives made from coconut, almonds, cashews, and other nuts and seeds. You can even find water kefir, which is tasty!

Where to find them: Find yogurt and kefir in the dairy section of your grocery store and often at farmers' markets, too. The challenge is finding quality brands, as most do not have many probiotic cultures in them and are loaded with sugars, artificial sweeteners, preservatives, flavorings, and colorings. Check labels: A good brand will have milk (or nondairy milk), cultures, and that's about it. Skip the low-fat and fat-free versions, as when manufacturers remove fat, they replace it with sugar and preservatives.

Prep tip: You can make kefir and yogurt at home without any special equipment. Either purchase kefir or yogurt starters, or use the method in this book with probiotic capsules. If using a starter, follow the instructions on the packet. And don't forget to save some of your kefir or yogurt to use as a starter for your next batch! If you have any extras, store in the refrigerator or freezer.

Note: If you are unaccustomed to consuming yogurt, kefir, or other fermented foods, start with a small amount. The influx of beneficial bacteria, if you aren't used to it, can lead to digestive symptoms like bloating, gas, and diarrhea. Begin with a few tablespoons, and work your way up to larger quantities.

Also note: In the following recipes, you can use nondairy kefir and yogurt and dairy kefir and yogurt interchangeably. Choosing yogurt over kefir will simply yield a thicker smoothie.

Basic Coconut Yogurt and Kefir

Energy Boost

Immunity Boost

Makes about 2 cups
Prep time: 5 minutes, plus
12 to 24 hours to ferment

For the coconut yogurt

1 (14-ounce) can coconut cream,
stirred (see tip)

2 probiotic capsules (or as many
capsules needed to reach 30 to
40 billion cultures)

1 tablespoon maple syrup or
coconut sugar

¾ teaspoon gelatin or
1 tablespoon coconut flour
(optional)

For the coconut kefir

1 (14-ounce) can full-fat coconut
milk, stirred (see tip)

2 probiotic capsules (or as many
capsules needed to reach 30 to
40 billion cultures)

1 tablespoon maple syrup or
coconut sugar

As you may have guessed by now, coconut milk is one of my favorite dairy-free alternatives. It's rich in beneficial fats and has a thick, creamy consistency that is perfect for smoothies. Its texture allows for a luxurious yogurt or kefir that resembles dairy, and it's very simple to make! Look for brands of coconut milk that have a simple ingredient list of coconut milk and water (xanthan gum or guar gum is fine, too). Any preservatives will prevent fermentation.

To make the coconut yogurt

1. In a small pot over medium heat, bring the coconut cream to a boil. Turn off the heat, and allow the cream to cool until the bowl is just warm to the touch. (If you happen to have a thermometer, anything less than 90°F is fine.) Transfer the cream to a small bowl or container with a lid.

2. Break open the probiotic capsules, and stir the powder and maple syrup into the coconut cream.

3. If using a bowl, cover the mixture with a tea towel. If using a container, place the lid on top but don't seal it. Allow the yogurt to ferment on the counter for 12 to 24 hours, until tangy. Fermentation time will depend on the time of year and temperature in your kitchen. You can facilitate fermentation by placing the bowl or container in a warm spot, like on top of the refrigerator, or in the oven with the oven light on only. Note: If you have a food dehydrator or an Instant Pot with a yogurt setting, you can also use those.

4. Once the yogurt is fermented to your liking, seal in a container or jar in the refrigerator. Save 2 to 3 tablespoons as a starter in a small container for your next batch. Consistency will thicken in the refrigerator slightly, and with subsequent batches. To enhance the thickness, blend the yogurt with ¾ teaspoon gelatin or 1 tablespoon coconut flour.

To make the coconut kefir

1. In a small pot over medium heat, bring the coconut milk to a boil. Turn off the heat, and allow the milk to cool until the bowl is just warm to the touch. (If you happen to have a thermometer, anything less than 90°F is fine.) Transfer the milk to a small bowl or container with a lid.
2. Break open the probiotic capsules, and stir the powder and maple syrup into the coconut milk.
3. If using a bowl, cover the mixture with a tea towel. If using a container, place the lid on top but don't seal it. Allow the kefir to ferment on the counter for 12 to 24 hours, until tangy. Fermentation time will depend on the time of year and temperature in your kitchen. You can facilitate fermentation by placing the bowl or container in a warm spot, like on top of the refrigerator, or in the oven with the oven light on only.
4. Once the kefir is fermented to your liking, seal in a container or jar in the refrigerator. Save 2 to 3 tablespoons as a starter in a small container for your next batch.

Substitute It! You can swap in any dairy-free milk in these recipes, but the result will be thinner than if you use coconut cream or milk. This is fine for kefir, though you may want to use the optional thickeners suggested in the yogurt instructions.

PER SERVING (¼ CUP) Calories: 189; Total Fat: 8 g; Sugars: 28 g; Carbohydrates: 29 g; Fiber: 0 g; Protein: 1 g

Strawberry Cheesecake Smoothie

Immunity Boost
Kid Friendly
Meal Swap

Makes 2 (14-ounce) servings
Prep time: 5 minutes

1¼ cups water or nondairy or
dairy milk of choice
½ cup plain, unsweetened
nondairy or dairy kefir or
yogurt of choice (store-bought
or homemade, page 70)
3 romaine lettuce leaves, torn
into pieces
2 cups frozen strawberries,
thawed 5 to 10 minutes for
easier blending
2 tablespoons ground almonds
1 teaspoon freshly squeezed
lemon juice
¼ teaspoon vanilla extract
Pinch salt

The tanginess of yogurt or kefir melds well with fruit to create cheesecake flavors. While the strawberries offer sweetness to balance sharper ferments, this recipe contains a boatload of vitamin C to support a healthy immune system. Cake in a glass—that's what I call a delicious breakfast.

1. In a blender, combine the water, kefir, lettuce, strawberries, almonds, lemon juice, vanilla, and salt. Blend until smooth, about 2 minutes, stopping the blender if needed to scrape down the sides so everything is fully incorporated.
2. Pour into two glasses and enjoy.

Taste Tip: If you have graham crackers or gingersnaps in the pantry, crumble them and sprinkle a tablespoon on top for added cheesecake flair.

PER SERVING Calories: 159; Total Fat: 6 g; Sugars: 13 g; Carbohydrates: 18 g; Fiber: 4 g; Protein: 6 g

Orange-Cream Popsicle Smoothie

Anti-Aging

Immunity Boost

Makes 2 (8-ounce) servings
Prep time: 5 minutes

---

1 cup water or nondairy or dairy
  milk of choice

½ cup plain, unsweetened
  nondairy or dairy yogurt or
  kefir of choice (store-bought
  or homemade, page 70)

2 large oranges, zested,
  peeled, and chopped into
  1-inch chunks

½ cup frozen mango

¼ cup frozen raspberries
  (optional)

¼ cup hemp seeds or
  2 tablespoons almond butter

Evoke childhood memories of summertime popsicles with this creamy orange smoothie. The zest and pith of oranges don't just enhance flavor; they offer health benefits, too. In addition to fiber and vitamin C, citrus peels contain flavonoids—special plant phytochemicals—called hesperidin and narirutin, which help prevent cardiovascular diseases, inflammation, cancer, and neurological decline. I recommend purchasing organic citrus whenever you are using the zest, as conventional peels contain pesticides and herbicides that can be damaging to your health (and won't rinse off).

1. In a blender, combine the water, yogurt, oranges, mango, raspberries (if using), and hemp seeds. Blend until smooth, about 2 minutes, stopping the blender if needed to scrape down the sides so everything is fully incorporated.
2. Pour into two glasses and enjoy.

✳ **Power Up!** Add a handful of dark leafy greens—dealer's choice—for additional antioxidants, fiber, and immune-boosting vitamins.

PER SERVING Calories: 275; Total Fat: 6 g; Sugars: 27 g; Carbohydrates: 32 g; Fiber: 5 g; Protein: 9 g

Sweet Potato Pie Power Surge

Anti-Inflammatory
Energy Boost
Immunity Boost

Makes 2 (12-ounce) servings
Prep time: 5 minutes

1 cup water or nondairy milk
   of choice
1 cup cooked, mashed sweet
   potatoes (about 2 medium
   potatoes—keep the skins on for
   extra nutrients)
½ cup plain, unsweetened nondairy kefir or yogurt of choice
   (store-bought or homemade,
   page 70)
½ frozen banana
¼ cup sunflower seed butter
Pinch ground nutmeg
Pinch salt
2 tablespoons pecans, chopped,
   for topping (optional)

Traditional sweet potato pie is loaded with flour, butter, cream, and sugar. In this health-ified, naturally sweetened, gluten-free, vegan version, sweet potatoes truly step into the spotlight. One of my favorite root vegetables, sweet potatoes are rich in beta-carotene, an antioxidant we convert to vitamin A for immunity, skin health, vision, and tissue repair. Additional evidence indicates they also have anti-tumor, anti-obesity, and anti-diabetic properties. Oh, and they're *yummy*—let's not forget that!

1. In a blender, combine the water, sweet potatoes, kefir, banana, sunflower seed butter, nutmeg, and salt. Blend until smooth, about 1 minute, stopping the blender if needed to scrape down the sides so everything is fully incorporated.
2. Pour into two glasses, sprinkle each with a tablespoon of pecans (if using), and enjoy.

Taste Tip: Add up to a teaspoon of ground cinnamon and fresh ginger to enhance the flavor.

PER SERVING Calories: 385; Total Fat: 16 g; Sugars: 15 g; Carbohydrates: 50 g; Fiber: 3 g; Protein: 13 g

Vegan Mango Lassi

Anti-Aging
Anti-Inflammatory

Makes 2 (8-ounce) servings
Prep time: 5 minutes

1 cup water
½ cup cashews, soaked for 2 to
6 hours and drained (see tip)
½ cup plain, unsweetened nondairy kefir or yogurt of choice
(store-bought or homemade,
page 70)
2 cups frozen mango
2 dates, pitted

I have been making variations of this smoothie for years now and always refer to it as "sunshine in a glass." If the weather is rainy and terrible, this smoothie will cheer you up. If the sun is out, it will enhance the joy you already feel. This one never fails to make me smile or go "Mmm."

1. In a blender, combine the water, cashews, kefir, mango, and dates. Blend until smooth, about 2 minutes, stopping the blender if needed to scrape down the sides so everything is fully incorporated.
2. Pour into two glasses and enjoy.

Substitute It! If you don't have the time to soak cashews, or you own a weak blender, use ¼ cup cashew butter instead. Also, once you are used to drinking kefir, you can swap it in for the cup of water, too.

PER SERVING Calories: 329; Total Fat: 14 g; Sugars: 32 g; Carbohydrates: 43 g; Fiber: 4 g; Protein: 10 g

Raspberry-Cream Decadence

Greens Lover

Meal Swap

Makes 2 (14-ounce) servings
Prep time: 5 minutes

1½ cups cashew milk

½ cup plain, unsweetened
coconut kefir or coconut
yogurt (store-bought or
homemade, page 70)

½ cup spinach, lightly packed
(see tip)

½ cup kale, lightly packed
(see tip)

1½ cups frozen raspberries

¼ cup ground pecans or almonds

Silky, thick cashew milk and coconut kefir or yogurt combine with raspberries and greens for a sweetly smooth green smoothie. I love raspberries here, though you could use any berry you fancy instead.

1. In a blender, combine the cashew milk, kefir, spinach, kale, raspberries, and pecans. Blend until smooth, about 2 minutes, stopping the blender if needed to scrape down the sides so everything is fully incorporated.
2. Pour into two glasses and enjoy.

Simplify It! Use spinach or kale only for easier prep.

PER SERVING Calories: 212; Total Fat: 9 g; Sugars: 22 g;
Carbohydrates: 31 g; Fiber: 7 g; Protein: 4 g

Creamy Lime and Spinach Smoothie

Anti-Inflammatory

Greens Lover

Makes 2 (10-ounce) servings
Prep time: 5 minutes

1 cup water or nondairy or dairy
   milk of choice

½ cup plain, unsweetened nondairy or dairy kefir or yogurt of
   choice (store-bought or homemade, page 70)

1 cup spinach, tightly packed

1 (4-inch) piece of cucumber, cut
   into 1-inch chunks

1 lime, zested, peeled, and cut into
   1-inch chunks

1 green apple, cored and cut into
   1-inch chunks

Handful of ice (optional)

This smoothie takes delightful tanginess to a whole new level with the blend of kefir/yogurt, whole lime, and green apple. There is no frozen fruit in here, making the smoothie thinner; this is easily corrected by throwing in some ice or a frozen banana for a touch of sweetness.

1. In a blender, combine the water, kefir, spinach, cucumber, lime, apple, and ice (if using). Blend until smooth, about 2 minutes, stopping the blender if needed to scrape down the sides so everything is fully incorporated.
2. Pour into two glasses and enjoy.

✳ **Power Up!** Add a tablespoon of freshly squeezed lemon juice and up to a teaspoon of freshly grated ginger for extra bite, along with more anti-inflammatory benefits.

PER SERVING Calories: 126; Total Fat: 1 g; Sugars: 18 g; Carbohydrates: 27 g; Fiber: 4 g; Protein: 5 g

Triple-Coconut Green Smoothie

Anti-Inflammatory

Energy Boost

Greens Lover

Meal Swap

Makes 2 (8-ounce) servings
Prep time: 5 minutes

1 cup full-fat coconut milk
½ cup plain, unsweetened
   coconut kefir or coconut yogurt
   (store-bought or homemade,
   page 70)
1 cup spinach, tightly packed
   (see tip)
1 frozen banana
2 tablespoons ground flaxseed
½ teaspoon vanilla extract
Pinch salt
2 tablespoons unsweetened,
   toasted shredded coconut,
   for topping

Coconut lovers unite! If you adore coconut as much as I do, you'll be glad to see that this recipe combines three different forms of it in one delicious green smoothie. Due to the amount of coconut, you'll likely feel satisfied from a small serving—and all those nutritious fats will help you absorb the vitamins in the greens, banana, and flaxseed.

1. In a blender, combine the coconut milk, kefir, spinach, banana, flaxseed, vanilla, and salt. Blend until smooth, about 2 minutes, stopping the blender if needed to scrape down the sides so everything is fully incorporated.
2. Pour into two glasses, top each with a tablespoon of shredded coconut, and enjoy.

Simplify It! If you want to keep your smoothie cream-colored and increase the coconut flavor, skip the greens or try a light-colored lettuce.

PER SERVING Calories: 450; Total Fat: 38 g; Sugars: 13 g; Carbohydrates: 27 g; Fiber: 9 g; Protein: 7 g

Probiotic Berry Slenderizer

Greens Lover

Heart Healthy

Meal Swap

Weight Loss

Makes 2 (14-ounce) servings
Prep time: 5 minutes

1½ cups water
½ cup nondairy kefir or yogurt of choice (store-bought or home-made, page 70)
2 cups mixed frozen berries of choice (see tip)
2 Swiss chard leaves, stemmed and torn into pieces
¾ cup spinach, tightly packed
¼ cup pumpkin seed butter

Combining yogurt and fruit enhances the effect of both, so you're getting a whopper of a smoothie here: This recipe mixes probiotic-rich kefir or yogurt with berries, and for an additional layer of benefits, packs in some leafy greens. The probiotics and fiber help support beneficial bacteria in the digestive tract, which aid digestion and eliminate excess waste, including cholesterol.

1. In a blender, combine the water, kefir, berries, chard, spinach, and pumpkin seed butter. Blend until smooth, about 2 minutes, stopping the blender if needed to scrape down the sides so everything is fully incorporated.
2. Pour into two glasses and enjoy.

Taste Tip: This recipe's sweetness will vary depending on the berries you choose. If the berries are tart, try adding a natural sweetener like dates, maple syrup, or honey.

PER SERVING Calories: 339; Total Fat: 19 g; Sugars: 19 g; Carbohydrates: 32 g; Fiber: 7 g; Protein: 12 g

Sweet Cherry-Vanilla Delight

Anti-Inflammatory

Heart Healthy

Makes 2 (8-ounce) servings
Prep time: 5 minutes

¾ cup water or nondairy or dairy milk of choice

½ cup plain, unsweetened nondairy or dairy kefir or yogurt of choice (store-bought or homemade, page 70)

1½ cups frozen, pitted cherries

¼ cup walnuts or 2 tablespoons nut/seed butter

1½ teaspoons vanilla extract

Pinch salt

As a child, I heard adults proclaim that certain fruits like cherries and strawberries were "like candy." This always seemed ridiculous to me, right up until my 20s: Fruit was fruit and candy was candy. When you're used to eating refined, sugary treats, you may find that fruit doesn't taste that sweet in comparison. But if you cut down your sugar intake, this can change. Now, I am happy to report that fruit *does* taste like candy—and I offer this smoothie as proof.

1. In a blender, combine the water, kefir, cherries, walnuts, vanilla, and salt. Blend until smooth, about 2 minutes, stopping the blender if needed to scrape down the sides so everything is fully incorporated.
2. Pour into two glasses and enjoy.

✴ **Power Up!** Use a teaspoon of ground cinnamon to enhance the sweetness, or add ¼ cup rolled oats for a satisfying breakfast.

PER SERVING Calories: 222; Total Fat: 9 g; Sugars: 21 g; Carbohydrates: 32 g; Fiber: 3 g; Protein: 7 g

Fiber-Full Stone Fruit and Cream Smoothie

Anti-Inflammatory

Greens Lover

Heart Healthy

Meal Swap

Makes 2 (14-ounce) servings
Prep time: 5 minutes

---

1 cup water or nondairy or dairy
    milk of choice

½ cup plain, unsweetened
    nondairy or dairy yogurt or
    kefir of choice (store-bought or
    homemade, page 70)

1 cup spinach, tightly packed

2 fresh peaches, pitted and
    chopped into 1-inch chunks

1 large, fresh nectarine,
    pitted and chopped into
    1-inch chunks

3 small apricots, pitted
    and halved

¼ cup sunflower seeds

The fact that stone fruit season is short and coincides with summer only makes it that much more delectable. Peaches, nectarines, and apricots are all rich in digestion-supportive, heart-healthy fiber, as well as immune-boosting vitamin C— and all are deliciously sweet!

1. In a blender, combine the water, yogurt, spinach, peaches, nectarine, apricots, and sunflower seeds. Blend until smooth, about 1 minute, stopping the blender if needed to scrape down the sides so everything is fully incorporated.
2. Pour into two glasses and enjoy.

Substitute It! Use any stone fruit in this recipe, including plums, pluots, cherries, mangos, or even fresh dates if you can get your hands on them.

PER SERVING Calories: 196; Total Fat: 5 g; Sugars: 29 g; Carbohydrates: 33 g; Fiber: 5 g; Protein: 8 g

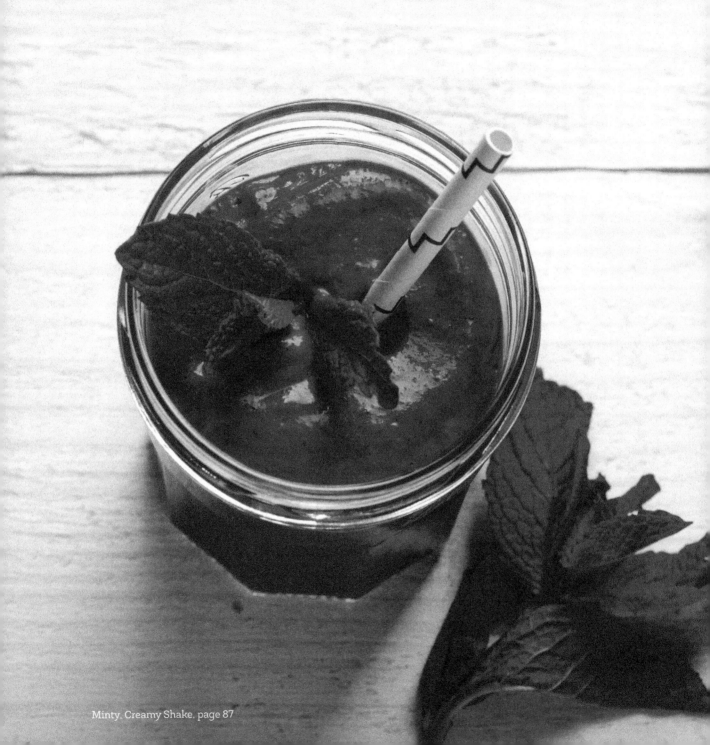

Minty, Creamy Shake, page 87

Chapter Six

Avocado

Avocado enthusiasts are flourishing in numbers around the world, and this isn't just due to a love of guacamole or avocado toast. The avocado's creamy texture is perfect for thickening smoothies, while its nutritional value is outstanding and can transform your smoothie into a satiating meal.

This amazing fruit contains high amounts of monounsaturated fats, particularly oleic acid, which is also found in olive oil. These fats help reduce inflammation throughout the body, balance blood sugar levels, and reduce cardiovascular risk.

Aside from their fats, avocados contain a broad spectrum of nutrients including fiber, protein, B vitamins (for energy, the brain, and your nervous system), and antioxidant vitamins A, C, and K. But that's not all: They also contain compounds that promote skin health and shield us from UV damage, protect against cancer, support eye health, and reduce arthritis symptoms. They truly are a comprehensive superfood!

Common forms: There are many different avocado varieties; one of the most common is Hass, also called the avocado pear or alligator pear.

Where to find them: Source avocados in the produce section of your grocery store. Selecting the perfect avocado can be tricky. Keep in mind that avocados continue to ripen after harvest and darken in color as they do. If an avocado looks ripe, give it a gentle squeeze. It should give in to pressure, but not collapse beneath your fingers. You can also check under the stem at the top: If the color beneath is green, the avocado is still good. If it's brown or black, it's overripe.

Prep tip: High concentrations of avocado nutrients are located in its pit and skin. So when peeling or scooping out the flesh, scrape as close to the skin as you can to obtain as many of those nutrients as possible. I tend not to freeze avocados because the texture is strange when they thaw, but this won't be a problem if you toss your frozen avocado straight into a blender.

Blueberry-Avocado Antioxidant Blast

Anti-Aging

Greens Lover

Heart Healthy

Meal Swap

Makes 2 (16-ounce) servings
Prep time: 5 minutes

1½ cups water or nondairy or
    dairy milk of choice
2 cups spinach, lightly packed
2 cups frozen blueberries
1 small avocado, peeled and pitted
¼ cup hemp seeds
2 dates, to sweeten (optional)

Combining antioxidant-rich blueberries with the nourishing fats and vitamins of avocados makes a fantastic smoothie for supporting cardiovascular health and keeping skin soft, smooth, and supple. If you can find wild blueberries, even better: Studies show they contain more antioxidants than cultivated ones because they need to tough it out in demanding environments.

1. In a blender, combine the water, spinach, blueberries, avocado, hemp seeds, and dates (if using). Blend until smooth, about 2 minutes, stopping the blender if needed to scrape down the sides so everything is fully incorporated.
2. Pour into two glasses and enjoy.

✳ **Power Up!** Add a teaspoon of matcha for more antioxidants.

PER SERVING Calories: 353; Total Fat: 19 g; Sugars: 15 g; Carbohydrates: 30 g; Fiber: 10 g; Protein: 7 g

Piña Colada Immunity Cocktail

Anti-Inflammatory Immunity Boost

Makes 2 (12-ounce) servings
Prep time: 5 minutes

¾ cup full-fat coconut milk
¾ cup water
1½ cups fresh or frozen pineapple
1 frozen banana
1 small avocado, peeled and pitted
1 orange, peeled and chopped into
   1-inch chunks
2 tablespoons almond butter

Now this is my version of a cocktail! In addition to the nutritious fats, immune-boosting vitamin C, and heart-healthy, blood sugar–balancing fiber, this smoothie features pineapple, which contains bromelain, an enzyme that aids in digestion while reducing inflammation and swelling. When possible, include the pineapple core in your smoothies, too, as that is where the highest concentration of bromelain lies.

1. In a blender, combine the coconut milk, water, pineapple, banana, avocado, orange, and almond butter. Blend until smooth, about 2 minutes, stopping the blender if needed to scrape down the sides so everything is fully incorporated.
2. Pour into two glasses and enjoy.

✷ **Power Up!** Transform this into a green smoothie by adding 1 cup of spinach, kale, or another green of your choice.

PER SERVING Calories: 607; Total Fat: 44 g; Sugars: 32 g; Carbohydrates: 56 g; Fiber: 15 g; Protein: 9 g

Minty, Creamy Shake

Greens Lover

Kid Friendly

Makes 2 (8-ounce) servings
Prep time: 5 minutes

1 cup nondairy or dairy milk
   of choice
1 cup spinach
1 avocado, peeled and pitted
4 to 6 fresh mint sprigs, stemmed,
   ½ teaspoon peppermint extract,
   or 2 to 3 drops food-grade peppermint essential oil
2 tablespoons cashew butter
1½ tablespoons raw honey or
   2 pitted dates

The Minty, Creamy Shake that inspired this one was created in the 1970s by a popular fast-food restaurant. This version skips the ice cream and artificial syrups and instead uses spinach for color; avocado, milk, and cashew butter for extra creaminess; and fresh mint for flavor. Yum!

1. In a blender, combine the milk, spinach, avocado, mint, cashew butter, and honey. Blend until smooth, about 2 minutes, stopping the blender if needed to scrape down the sides so everything is fully incorporated. Taste, and add more sweetener if necessary.
2. Pour into two glasses and enjoy.

✳ **Power Up!** Pour in ½ cup plain, unsweetened nondairy or dairy yogurt or kefir of your choice (store-bought or home-made, page 70) for extra creaminess and probiotic benefits, or sprinkle cacao nibs on top for a hit of dark chocolate.

PER SERVING Calories: 332; Total Fat: 24 g; Sugars: 13 g;
Carbohydrates: 27 g; Fiber: 8 g; Protein: 6 g

Creamy Avocado, Strawberry, and Mint Smoothie

. . . .

Anti-Inflammatory

Greens Lover

Meal Swap

Makes 2 (14-ounce) servings
Prep time: 5 minutes

1½ cups water or nondairy or
   dairy milk of choice
1¼ cups spinach or lettuce, lightly
   packed (see tip)
2 cups frozen strawberries,
   thawed 5 to 10 minutes for
   easier blending
1 avocado, peeled and pitted
4 fresh mint sprigs, stemmed
2 tablespoons sunflower
   seed butter

Here's a refreshing and fruity smoothie with creamy avocado providing some extra "oomph." For additional anti-inflammatory, immune-boosting vitamin C and hydration, slice up some cucumber (don't peel off the skin!) and toss it into the blender, too.

1. In a blender, combine the water, spinach, strawberries, avocado, mint, and sunflower seed butter. Blend until smooth, about 2 minutes, stopping the blender if needed to scrape down the sides so everything is fully incorporated.
2. Pour into two glasses and enjoy.

Simplify It! If you're not in the mood for greens, just leave 'em out.

PER SERVING Calories: 298; Total Fat: 21 g; Sugars: 9 g; Carbohydrates: 27 g; Fiber: 10 g; Protein: 6 g

Avocado, Walnut, and Coconut Get-Up-and-Go

Energy Boost

Greens Lover

Heart Healthy

Meal Swap

Makes 2 (10-ounce) servings
Prep time: 5 minutes

¾ **cup full-fat coconut milk**
¾ **cup water**
⅓ **cup walnuts**
1 cup spinach, lightly packed
1 avocado, peeled and pitted
1 frozen banana (see tip)

If you find it tough to get going in the morning, this smoothie may be just the ticket. The avocado and coconut fats will keep you fueled for hours, and walnuts are nutritional powerhouses: They've been shown to reduce blood pressure and cholesterol, support a healthy weight, and delay and prevent cognitive decline.

1. In a blender, combine the coconut milk, water, walnuts, spinach, avocado, and banana. Blend until smooth, about 2 minutes, stopping the blender if needed to scrape down the sides so everything is fully incorporated.
2. Pour into two glasses and enjoy.

Substitute It! Swap ¾ cup of any frozen berry for the banana in this recipe.

PER SERVING Calories: 548; Total Fat: 49 g; Sugars: 11 g; Carbohydrates: 29 g; Fiber: 11 g; Protein: 8 g

Avocado-Herb Fest

Greens Lover

Makes 2 (12-ounce) servings
Prep time: 5 minutes

1½ cups water or nondairy or
    dairy milk of choice
1 cup fresh parsley, lightly packed
    (see tip)
8 fresh mint sprigs, stemmed
1½ cups frozen mango
1 avocado, peeled and pitted
2 tablespoons flaxseed

Herbs are often used as a garnish and plucked off the plate or pushed to the side. Put simply: They don't always receive the adoration they deserve. This smoothie brings herbs to the forefront. In fact, they're the only greens in this recipe—so they're the star of the show!

1. In a blender, combine the water, parsley, mint, mango, avocado, and flaxseed. Blend until smooth, about 2 minutes, stopping the blender if needed to scrape down the sides so everything is fully incorporated.
2. Pour into two glasses and enjoy.

Substitute It! Try switching out half or all of the parsley for fresh cilantro, or add a handful of fresh basil.

PER SERVING Calories: 307; Total Fat: 19 g; Sugars: 17 g; Carbohydrates: 34 g; Fiber: 14 g; Protein: 7 g

Calming Avocado-Lavender Smoothie

Anti-Inflammatory
Immunity Boost

Makes 2 (8-ounce) servings
Prep time: 5 minutes

1 cup water or nondairy or dairy
  milk of choice
1 cup frozen blueberries
1 avocado, peeled and pitted
2 tablespoons almond butter
½ teaspoon culinary lavender
  (see tip)
½ teaspoon freshly squeezed
  lemon juice

You might be familiar with using lavender-scented beauty products but have less experience eating it. However, culinary lavender makes a lovely addition to smoothies. It's calming to the nervous system, helps relieve anxiety and pain, and is even known to improve mood and sleep quality. Its floral flavor pairs well with blueberries, but you can use other types of berries instead, or frozen bananas.

1. In a blender, combine the water, blueberries, avocado, almond butter, lavender, and lemon juice. Blend until smooth, about 1 minute, stopping the blender if needed to scrape down the sides so everything is fully incorporated.
2. Pour into two glasses and enjoy.

Taste Tip: Culinary lavender can have a strong flavor, so start with the amount listed here, and if you really love it, move up to 1 teaspoon.

PER SERVING Calories: 284; Total Fat: 23 g; Sugars: 8 g; Carbohydrates: 21 g; Fiber: 9 g; Protein: 6 g

Seductive Green Goddess

Greens Lover

Meal Swap

Weight Loss

Makes 2 (10-ounce) servings
Prep time: 5 minutes

1½ cups water or nondairy or
dairy milk of choice
1 cup spinach, tightly packed
1 avocado, peeled and pitted
1 pear, chopped into 1-inch
chunks (see tip)
¼ cup tahini
1 tablespoon honey
1 teaspoon freshly squeezed
lemon juice

Classic green goddess dressing typically includes herbs, mayonnaise, sour cream, garlic, and some form of acidity. While the name may evoke an ethereal, floating free spirit, the dressing was in fact created in the 1920s to honor a popular play of the same title and its lead actor. This smoothie version is sweeter than the dressing but retains its creaminess and pale green beauty.

1. In a blender, combine the water, spinach, avocado, pear, tahini, honey, and lemon juice. Blend until smooth, about 2 minutes, stopping the blender if needed to scrape down the sides so everything is fully incorporated.
2. Pour into two glasses and enjoy.

Substitute It! For a slightly sweeter and thicker texture, swap in 1 frozen banana for the pear.

PER SERVING Calories: 399; Total Fat: 30 g; Sugars: 16 g; Carbohydrates: 34 g; Fiber: 11 g; Protein: 8 g

Avocado-Almond-Banana Pump-Up

Energy Boost

Kid Friendly

Meal Swap

Makes 2 (14-ounce) servings

Prep time: 5 minutes

2¼ cups nondairy or dairy milk
   of choice

2 tablespoons almond butter

1 banana, peeled and chopped

1 avocado, peeled and pitted

2 dates, pitted and soaked in
   warm water to soften

¼ cup crushed ice (optional),
   plus more as needed

Looking for a satisfying smoothie with rich, nutty flavor as well as protein and fat to get you through the morning? This is the perfect breakfast with its tempting, sweet flavor and impressive staying power. If purchasing almond butter, remember to choose unsweetened to keep sugars low.

1. In a blender, combine the milk, almond butter, banana, avocado, dates, and ice (if using). Blend for 30 seconds.
2. Stop and use a spatula to scrape down the sides. Blend for 30 seconds to 1 minute more on high, until smooth. Blend in a little water or ice as needed to adjust consistency.
3. Pour into two glasses and enjoy.

✳ **Power Up!** Add 2 teaspoons of antioxidant-rich cocoa powder for a chocolate-almond-banana smoothie.

PER SERVING Calories: 413; Total Fat: 29 g; Sugars: 13 g; Carbohydrates: 33 g; Fiber: 12 g; Protein: 9 g

Avocado, Citrus, and Pumpkin Seed Energizer

Energy Boost

Meal Swap

Makes 2 (14-ounce) servings
Prep time: 5 minutes

1½ cups unsweetened or freshly
squeezed orange juice, plus
more as needed

¼ cup raw, unsalted
pumpkin seeds

1 avocado, peeled and pitted

¾ cup unsweetened nondairy or
dairy milk of choice

¼ cup ice (optional), plus more
as needed

Citrus and pumpkin seeds add a sweetly nutty flavor and a healthy boost of essential energizing micro- and macronutrients like vitamin C, protein, iron, manganese, and zinc. Be sure to use raw, unsalted, shelled pumpkin seeds (also called pepitas) and no-sugar-added orange juice.

1. In a blender, combine the orange juice and pumpkin seeds. Process with 20 (one-second) pulses to chop the seeds, then blend on high for 30 seconds.
2. Add the avocado, milk, and ice (if using). Blend for 30 seconds to 1 minute more on high, until smooth. Blend in a little juice or ice as needed to adjust consistency.
3. Pour into two glasses and enjoy.

✳ **Power Up!** Add ¾ cup of plain, unsweetened nondairy or dairy yogurt or kefir of your choice (store-bought or homemade, page 70) alongside the avocado for smoothness and additional protein.

PER SERVING Calories: 328; Total Fat: 23 g; Sugars: 16 g; Carbohydrates: 30 g; Fiber: 8 g; Protein: 8 g

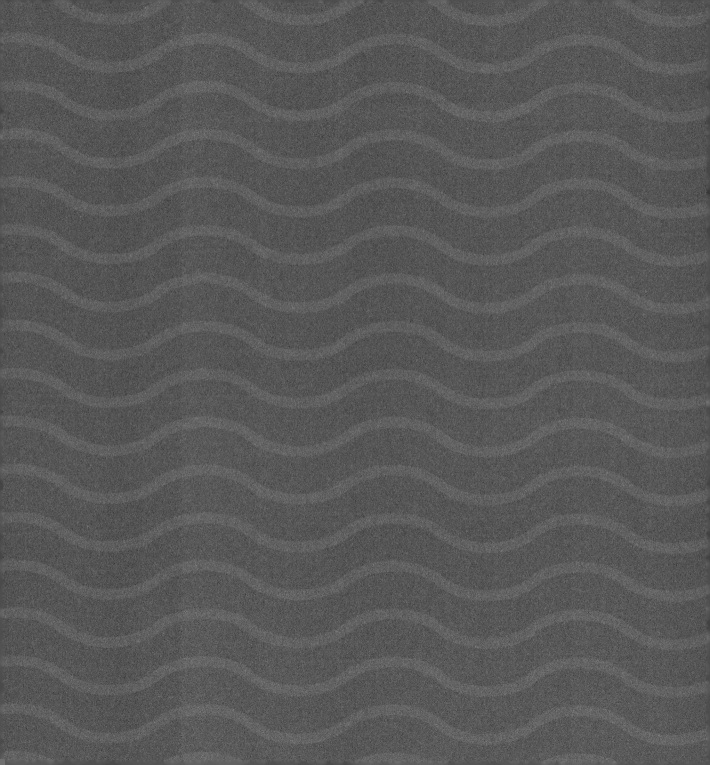

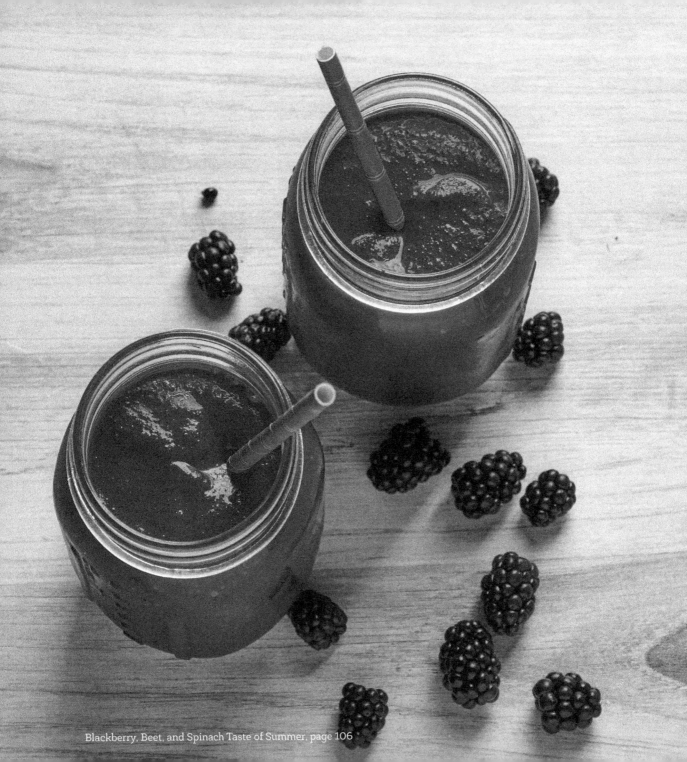
Blackberry, Beet, and Spinach Taste of Summer, page 106

Chapter Seven

Beets

They're not just for borscht! Beets—also known as beetroot—thrive in cold and hardy climates and are gaining recognition as a superfood for their nutritional benefits, availability, and low cost. They are a striking source of antioxidants. One unique group of antioxidants in beets is called betalains, which hinders the enzymes that trigger inflammation and encourages our bodies' natural detoxification processes. (These plant pigments are also responsible for the beet's vivid colors.) Beet compounds have also been studied for their ability to balance blood sugar levels, encourage weight loss, stamp out oxidative stress that destroys our tissues, lower blood pressure, and improve blood vessel function. They may even shore up brain function and reduce our cancer risk. On top of all this, their sweet flavor tastes wonderful in smoothies. You simply can't "beet" all that.

Common forms: Fresh beets are available in a rainbow of colors, including white, yellow, orange, pink, red, purple, and striped. You can also find beet juice—read labels to ensure the juice contains no added sugars or fillers—and concentrated beet powders, which tend to be expensive. Beet juices lack fiber and are higher in calories, so that is something to keep in mind (you may want to use less in your smoothies).

Where to find them: Fresh beets are available in the produce section of your grocery store or at farmers' markets. Look for smooth and firm beets free of blemishes or shriveled bits. Beet juice will be in the juice aisle, or in a refrigerated section if your shop makes fresh-pressed juice.

Prep tip: You can use raw, roasted, or steamed beets in smoothies. However, some find that raw beets taste too "earthy," so cooking or roasting enhances their natural sweetness. When grated or chopped small, raw beets are easy to prep and blend—you also avoid long cooking times.

If the beet greens are still attached, save them to use in other smoothies or stir-fries.

Sweet Beet and Orange Treat

Energy Boost

Weight Loss

Makes 2 (12-ounce) servings
Prep time: 5 minutes

2 cups unsweetened or freshly
squeezed orange juice

1 cup unsweetened nondairy or
dairy milk of choice

1 cup chopped or ½ cup grated red
or golden beets

2 tablespoons tahini

1 teaspoon cardamom seeds
(see tip)

¼ cup crushed ice (optional)

Beets' sweet and earthy flavor pairs well with citrus. While the recipe calls for raw beets—peeled and chopped—you can also use cooked and well-drained beets for a smoother texture to your smoothie.

1. In a blender, combine the orange juice, milk, beets, tahini, cardamom, and ice (if using). Blend until smooth, about 2 minutes, stopping the blender if needed to scrape down the sides so everything is fully incorporated.

2. Pour into two glasses and enjoy.

✳ **Power Up!** Replace the cardamom seeds with 1 tablespoon of freshly grated ginger or turmeric for an anti-inflammatory, antioxidant boost.

PER SERVING Calories: 284; Total Fat: 12 g; Sugars: 28 g; Carbohydrates: 39 g; Fiber: 5 g; Protein: 7 g

Tropical Beet-the-Bloat Smoothie

Immunity Boost

Kid Friendly

Makes 2 (16-ounce) servings

Prep time: 5 minutes

2 cups unsweetened coconut
water, plus more if needed

½ cup full-fat coconut milk

1 cup chopped or ½ cup grated red
or golden beets

1 cup unsweetened chopped
pineapple

1 cup chopped papaya, peeled
and seeded

¼ cup almond butter

Feeling bloated? This sweet beet smoothie can help with enzyme-rich fruits including pineapple and papaya. Adding unsweetened coconut water helps hydration, too. With a tropical, sweet flavor, this is sure to become a family favorite.

1. In a blender, combine the coconut water, coconut milk, beets, pineapple, papaya, and almond butter. Blend until smooth, about 2 minutes, stopping the blender if needed to scrape down the sides so everything is fully incorporated. Add more coconut water if needed to adjust the thickness.
2. Pour into two glasses and enjoy.

✴ **Power Up!** Transform this into a green smoothie by adding 1 cup of your favorite greens.

PER SERVING Calories: 520; Total Fat: 35 g; Sugars: 39 g; Carbohydrates: 53 g; Fiber: 7 g; Protein: 8 g

Glowing Skin Beet and Raspberry Smoothie

Anti-Aging

Anti-Inflammatory

Makes 2 (14-ounce) servings
Prep time: 5 minutes

1½ cups water or nondairy or dairy milk of choice

1 cup unsweetened apple juice

1 cup chopped or ½ cup grated red beets

1 cup fresh or frozen unsweetened raspberries

¼ cup almond butter

¼ cup crushed ice (optional)

At once sweet and tangy, this smoothie will please your palate while giving your skin a healthy glow. It's packed with antioxidants like vitamins A and C, so drinking this smoothie on a regular basis encourages your body to promote cellular repair and produce radiant skin.

1. In a blender, combine the water, apple juice, beets, raspberries, almond butter, and ice (if using). Blend until smooth, about 2 minutes, stopping the blender if needed to scrape down the sides so everything is fully incorporated.

2. Pour into two glasses and enjoy.

✳ **Power Up!** Green tea is also great for glowing skin. For an extra boost of antioxidants, replace the apple juice with freshly brewed and cooled unsweetened green tea, or add a tablespoon of matcha powder.

PER SERVING Calories: 330; Total Fat: 20 g; Sugars: 25 g; Carbohydrates: 37 g; Fiber: 7 g; Protein: 7 g

Beet and Apple Blood Sugar Balancer

....

Anti-Inflammatory

Energy Boost

Makes 2 (12-ounce) servings
Prep time: 5 minutes

1½ cups water or nondairy or
   dairy milk of choice
1 cup unsweetened apple juice
½ cup plain, unsweetened nondairy or dairy yogurt or kefir
   (store-bought or homemade,
   page 70)
1 cup chopped or ½ cup grated
   red beets
2 apples, peeled, cored,
   and chopped

Apples and beets are both high in fiber, so they can help keep blood sugar in check despite their sweet flavor. This smoothie contains plenty of fiber, and its sweet and mellow flavor makes it an ideal snack when your energy dips and you need a little boost.

1. In a blender, combine the water, apple juice, yogurt, beets, and apples. Blend until smooth, 2 to 3 minutes, stopping the blender if needed to scrape down the sides so everything is fully incorporated.
2. Pour into two glasses and enjoy.

✳ **Power Up!** For even more blood sugar control, add up to 1 teaspoon of ground cinnamon.

PER SERVING Calories: 255; Total Fat: 1 g; Sugars: 48 g; Carbohydrates: 58 g; Fiber: 7 g; Protein: 6 g

Beet, Cherry, Lime, and Mint Immunity Boost

Anti-Inflammatory

Greens Lover

Heart Healthy

Immunity Boost

Makes 2 (12-ounce) servings
Prep time: 5 minutes

1 cup unsweetened tart cherry juice (see tip)

1 cup spinach, lightly packed

1 cup chopped or ½ cup grated red beets

1½ cups fresh or frozen Bing cherries, pitted and halved

¼ cup fresh mint leaves

Zest and juice of 1 lime

¼ cup crushed ice (optional)

Beets and cherries are both sweet, but when you combine them with the acidity of lime juice and the herbaceous flavor of mint, the result is a balanced and flavorful smoothie. Mint is also great when you have a cold, so this antioxidant-rich smoothie is a must-have if you're feeling under the weather.

1. In a blender, combine the cherry juice, spinach, beets, cherries, mint, lime zest and juice, and ice (if using). Blend until smooth, 2 to 3 minutes, stopping the blender if needed to scrape down the sides so everything is fully incorporated.
2. Pour into two glasses and enjoy.

Substitute It! You can normally find unsweetened tart cherry juice at your local health food store. If you're unable to locate it, simply substitute 1 cup of unsweetened apple or white grape juice.

PER SERVING Calories: 154; Total Fat: 1 g; Sugars: 22 g; Carbohydrates: 37 g; Fiber: 3 g; Protein: 3 g

Beet, Orange, Carrot, and Banana Anti-Aging Mix

Anti-Aging
Anti-Inflammatory
Immunity Boost

Makes 2 (16-ounce) servings
Prep time: 5 minutes

2 cups unsweetened orange juice
1 cup chopped or ½ cup grated red or golden beets
2 oranges, peeled and broken into sections
2 carrots, peeled and finely chopped or grated
1 frozen banana
¼ cup hemp seeds

Combining the lovely citrus flavor of sweet beets and carrots with the mellow, smooth taste of bananas, this is a balanced smoothie that isn't too earthy from the beets, nor is it overly sweet. It's also packed with antioxidants to support cellular health and rejuvenation.

1. In a blender, combine the orange juice, beets, oranges, carrots, banana, and hemp seeds. Blend until smooth, 2 to 3 minutes, stopping the blender if needed to scrape down the sides so everything is fully incorporated.
2. Pour into two glasses and enjoy.

☀ **Power Up!** Boost the anti-inflammatory and antioxidant benefits of this recipe by adding 1 tablespoon of freshly grated ginger.

PER SERVING Calories: 426; Total Fat: 6 g; Sugars: 55 g; Carbohydrates: 74 g; Fiber: 10 g; Protein: 9 g

Hidden Veggie Beet Smoothie

Greens Lover

Kid Friendly

Makes 2 (16-ounce) servings
Prep time: 5 minutes

1½ cups unsweetened apple or
  pear juice
1 cup finely chopped spinach
  (see tip)
1 cup finely chopped
  kale, stemmed
½ cup fresh or frozen Bing cherries, peeled, pitted, and finely
  chopped (see tip)
½ cup plain, unsweetened nondairy or dairy yogurt or kefir of
  choice (store-bought or homemade, page 70)
1 cup chopped or ½ cup grated
  red beets
1 pear, peeled, cored, and
  finely chopped
¼ cup almond butter
Pinch ground nutmeg
¼ crushed ice (optional)

Have picky eaters who don't love their greens? Incorporating them into a smoothie is a lightly sweet, delicious way to enjoy them. The trick is in the blending: Blend on high for as long as it takes for those veggies to disappear!

1. In a blender, combine the apple juice, spinach, kale, cherries, yogurt, beets, pear, almond butter, nutmeg, and ice (if using). Blend until smooth, about 3 minutes, stopping the blender if needed to scrape down the sides so everything is fully incorporated.
2. Pour into two glasses and enjoy.

Simplify It! Use frozen cherries and frozen spinach, which will save the time required to wash, chop, and pit.

PER SERVING Calories: 451; Total Fat: 20 g; Sugars: 43 g; Carbohydrates: 61 g; Fiber: 7 g; Protein: 12 g

Blackberry, Beet, and Spinach
Taste of Summer

Energy Boost

Greens Lover

Weight Loss

Makes 2 (16-ounce) servings

Prep time: 5 minutes

---

1 cup unsweetened 100 percent
   cranberry juice

2 cups chopped fresh spinach

2 cups fresh or frozen
   blackberries

1 cup chopped or ½ cup grated
   red beets

¼ cup sunflower seed butter

Blackberries are in season in the mid to late summer; however, using frozen blackberries to add sweetness to this antioxidant-filled smoothie will allow you to enjoy their taste all year long!

1. In a blender, combine the cranberry juice, spinach, blackberries, beets, and sunflower seed butter. Blend until smooth, about 3 minutes, stopping the blender if needed to scrape down the sides so everything is fully incorporated.

2. Pour into two glasses and enjoy.

✳ **Power Up!** To round out this smoothie and add probiotic benefits, use ½ cup plain, unsweetened nondairy or dairy yogurt or kefir of your choice (store-bought or homemade, page 70).

PER SERVING Calories: 332; Total Fat: 16 g; Sugars: 18 g;
Carbohydrates: 42 g; Fiber: 10 g; Protein: 11 g

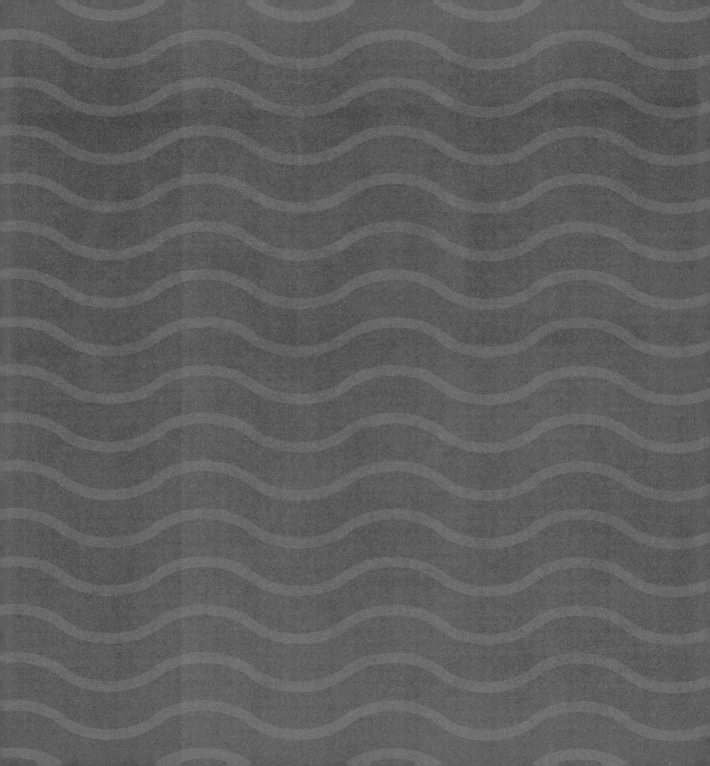

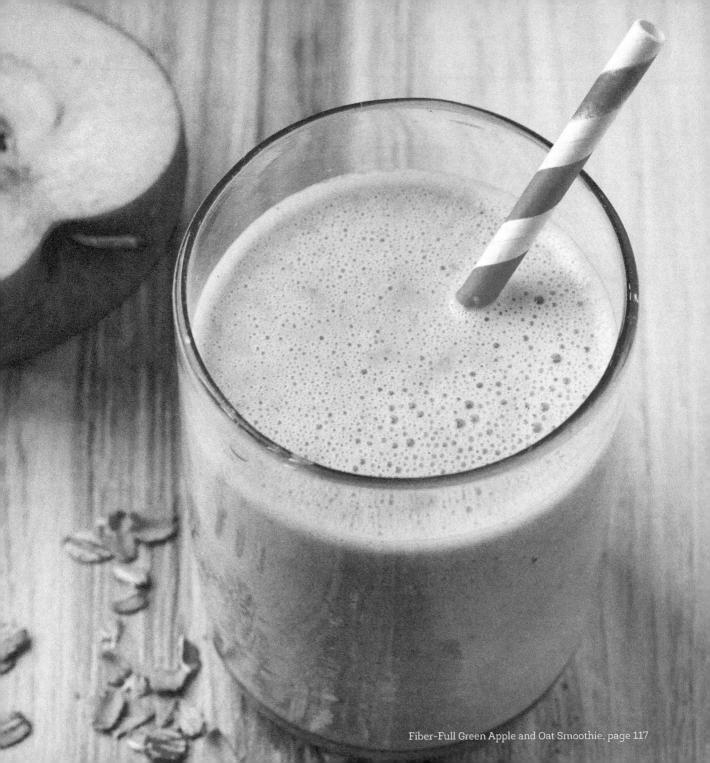

Fiber-Full Green Apple and Oat Smoothie, page 117

Chapter Eight

Oats

I love the thick texture oats supply to smoothies. They also contain nutrients like B vitamins that lift energy levels and minerals that balance blood sugar, but these are all fringe benefits alongside their principal staying power: fiber. There are two types of fiber: soluble, which swells up in water and allows food to pass slowly through the digestive tract, leading to better nutrient absorption and feeling full; and insoluble, a fiber that passes through the digestive tract without breaking down, but is just as important because it bulks up our stool and prevents constipation.

Oats contain both types of fiber, but they are an especially good source of a soluble fiber called beta-glucans. Oat beta-glucans move slowly through the digestive tract, where they are fully digested and feed the beneficial bacteria in the gut, as well as increase our satiety. They also lower blood sugar levels and cholesterol, enhance the immune system, and inhibit tumor growth. Oat consumption is linked with weight loss, a reduced risk of cardiovascular disease and diabetes, and better digestive health. If you're tired of oatmeal for breakfast, eat your oats in smoothies instead! And yes, you can eat them raw.

Common forms: From thickest texture to thinnest: steel cut, old fashioned/rolled, and quick-cooking/instant.

Where to find them: Locate oats in the cereal aisle or bulk section of the grocery store.

Prep tip: Rolled oats are my go-to for smoothies, though you can also choose quick-cooking/instant oats for smoother blending. If gluten intolerance is an issue, purchase certified gluten-free oats.

Blueberry Crumble Antioxidant Support

Energy Boost
Heart Healthy

Makes 2 (10-ounce) servings
Prep time: 5 minutes

¼ **cup rolled oats**
2 **cups nondairy or dairy milk**
of choice
2 **cups fresh or frozen blueberries**
½ **cup plain, unsweetened**
nondairy or dairy yogurt or
kefir of choice (store-bought or
homemade, page 70)
½ **teaspoon vanilla extract**
¼ **teaspoon ground nutmeg**
¼ **cup crushed ice (optional)**

This smoothie tastes like dessert in a cup, but it's actually reasonably low in sugar and bursting with the flavors of blueberry and vanilla. The oats add a nice, hearty touch to the smoothie, so it makes a great meal replacement packed with antioxidants.

1. Put the oats in a blender. Process with 20 to 30 (one-second) pulses, until finely ground.
2. Add the milk, blueberries, yogurt, vanilla, nutmeg, and ice (if using), and blend until smooth, 2 to 3 minutes, stopping the blender if needed to scrape down the sides so everything is fully incorporated.
3. Pour into two glasses and enjoy.

⋇ **Power Up!** Cinnamon and ginger both add a lot to the flavor of this smoothie, and increase its superfood status. Add ½ teaspoon ground cinnamon and ½ teaspoon ground ginger or 1 tablespoon grated fresh ginger to give this smoothie more flavor and nutrition.

PER SERVING Calories: 256; Total Fat: 8 g; Sugars: 19 g; Carbohydrates: 35 g; Fiber: 7 g; Protein: 9 g

Oatmeal-Raisin Breakfast Smoothie

Energy Boost
Heart Healthy
Kid Friendly

Makes 2 (10-ounce) servings
Prep time: 5 minutes

½ cup rolled oats
2 cups unsweetened nondairy or
  dairy milk of choice
1 frozen banana
¼ cup almond butter or sunflower
  seed butter
¼ cup raisins
2 dates, soaked, pitted, and
  finely chopped
½ teaspoon vanilla extract
¼ teaspoon ground nutmeg

Do you like oatmeal cookies? This smoothie is a riff on that, with oatmeal cookie flavor and just a hint of nutmeg. It's full of fiber and gets its sweetness from soaked dates and a banana. Although it resembles a dessert, this is the perfect breakfast smoothie.

1. Put the oats in a blender. Process with 20 to 30 (one-second) pulses, until finely ground.
2. Add the milk, banana, almond butter, raisins, dates, vanilla, and nutmeg, and blend until smooth, 2 to 3 minutes, stopping the blender if needed to scrape down the sides so everything is fully incorporated.
3. Pour into two glasses and enjoy.

✳ **Power Up!** Want it to taste even more like a cookie and increase its superfood status? Add ½ teaspoon freshly ground cinnamon.

PER SERVING Calories: 479; Total Fat: 23 g; Sugars: 24 g; Carbohydrates: 59 g; Fiber: 7 g; Protein: 13 g

Sunbutter, Apple, and Oatmeal Vitamin Boost

Energy Boost

Heart Healthy

Makes 2 (10-ounce) servings
Prep time: 5 minutes

½ cup rolled oats
1 cup unsweetened apple juice
2 tablespoons unsweetened sunbutter
1 apple, peeled, cored, and finely chopped
¼ teaspoon ground nutmeg
1½ cups nondairy or dairy milk of choice
½ cup plain, unsweetened non-dairy or dairy yogurt or kefir of choice (store-bought or home-made, page 70)
½ teaspoon vanilla extract
¼ cup crushed ice (optional)

Made with sunflower seeds, sunbutter is an excellent source of vitamins, including the heart-healthy antioxidant vitamin E, B vitamins for energy, plus magnesium for bone health. Sunbutter is also a good source of healthy fat and fiber, and contributes a deliciously nutty flavor to this smoothie.

1. Put the oats in a blender. Process with 20 to 30 (one-second) pulses, until finely ground.
2. Add the apple juice, sunbutter, apple, and nutmeg, and blend until smooth, about 2 minutes.
3. Add the milk, yogurt, vanilla, and ice (if using), and blend for another minute, or until smooth, stopping the blender if needed to scrape down the sides so everything is fully incorporated.
4. Pour into two glasses and enjoy.

Taste Tip: Ground ginger will add lots of flavor to this already tasty smoothie. Add ½ teaspoon in the second step.

PER SERVING Calories: 395; Total Fat: 15 g; Sugars: 30 g; Carbohydrates: 54 g; Fiber: 7 g; Protein: 12 g

Hearty Berry-Granola Crunch

Anti-Inflammatory

Greens Lover

Meal Swap

Makes 2 (12-ounce) servings
Prep time: 5 minutes

1 cup nondairy or dairy milk
of choice

1 cup unsweetened apple juice

½ cup plain, unsweetened nondairy or dairy yogurt or kefir of
choice (store-bought or homemade, page 70)

1 cup chopped fresh spinach

2 cups frozen unsweetened
mixed berries

¼ cup hemp seeds or nuts/seeds
of choice

4 tablespoons unsweetened
granola, divided

Adding granola to this recipe—both blended into the smoothie and as a garnish—produces a nice crunch. This works especially well for a smoothie bowl you eat with a spoon. At the same time, the smoothie is packed with antioxidant-rich berries and some hidden greens for a punch of extra nutrition.

1. In a blender, combine the milk, apple juice, yogurt, spinach, berries, hemp seeds, and 3 tablespoons of granola. Blend until smooth, about 2 minutes, stopping the blender if needed to scrape down the sides so everything is fully incorporated.

2. Pour into two glasses or bowls, garnish with the remaining tablespoon of granola, and enjoy.

Taste Tip: If you would prefer a sweeter smoothie, add a few drops of liquid stevia or one date, soaked in warm water and finely chopped, to the blender.

PER SERVING Calories: 375; Total Fat: 10 g; Sugars: 30 g; Carbohydrates: 42 g; Fiber: 7 g; Protein: 10 g

Cherry, Coconut, and Oat Temptation

Energy Boost

Immunity Boost

Kid Friendly

Makes 2 (12-ounce) servings
Prep time: 5 minutes

½ cup rolled oats

2 cups unsweetened coconut water, chilled or frozen into cubes

¼ cup full-fat coconut milk

2 cups fresh or frozen Bing cherries, pitted and halved

2 tablespoons ground flaxseed

¼ cup crushed ice (optional)

Coconut water and coconut milk add creaminess and an unmistakable tropical accent to this sweet smoothie. Meanwhile, the cherries are especially high in antioxidants, and coconut water is both hydrating and energizing, creating a tempting yet healthy smoothie for kids of all ages.

1. Put the oats in a blender. Process with 20 to 30 (one-second) pulses, until finely ground.
2. Add the coconut water, coconut milk, cherries, flaxseed, and ice (if using), and blend until smooth, 2 to 3 minutes, stopping the blender if needed to scrape down the sides so everything is fully incorporated.
3. Pour into two glasses and enjoy.

Substitute It! Bump up the probiotic benefits and increase tanginess by spooning ¼ cup plain, unsweetened coconut yogurt or kefir of choice (store-bought or homemade, page 70) into the blender.

PER SERVING Calories: 364; Total Fat: 14 g; Sugars: 35 g; Carbohydrates: 57 g; Fiber: 10 g; Protein: 8 g

Lettuce at 'Em Oat Smoothie

Energy Boost

Greens Lover

Immunity Boost

Makes 2 (14-ounce) servings

Prep time: 5 minutes

½ cup rolled oats

2 cups unsweetened apple
    juice, chilled

2 cups chopped romaine lettuce

2 apples, peeled, cored, and finely
    chopped or grated

¼ cup fresh parsley

Juice of 1 lemon

¼ cup crushed ice (optional)

Get your greens in this herbaceous oat smoothie that is super for detoxification. This one's not sweet: It's herbal and oaty, but is a great energy booster packing in high doses of vitamin C and antioxidants. Think of it as salad in a cup, in the best possible way.

1. Put the oats in a blender. Pulse with 20 to 30 (one-second) pulses, until finely ground.
2. Add the apple juice, lettuce, apples, parsley, lemon juice, and ice (if using), and blend until smooth, 2 to 3 minutes, stopping the blender if needed to scrape down the sides so everything is fully incorporated.
3. Pour into two glasses and enjoy.

Substitute It! You can substitute any greens here or mix up the lettuce. For example, try 1 cup of red lettuce and 1 cup of romaine.

PER SERVING Calories: 323; Total Fat: 2 g; Sugars: 52 g; Carbohydrates: 76 g; Fiber: 8 g; Protein: 4 g

Fiber-Full Green Apple and Oat Smoothie

Energy Boost

Heart Healthy

Immunity Boost

Makes 2 (14-ounce) servings

Prep time: 5 minutes

½ cup rolled oats

¼ cup chopped walnuts

2 cups unsweetened apple juice

½ cup plain, unsweetened non-dairy or dairy yogurt or kefir of choice (store-bought or home-made, page 70)

2 green apples, peeled, cored, and finely chopped or grated

¼ teaspoon ground nutmeg

½ teaspoon vanilla extract

¼ cup crushed ice (optional)

Granny Smith apples make the perfect green apple selection for this tart-sweet smoothie. You can also try a sweet-tart apple variety like Honeycrisp. Packed with fiber, this is a filling smoothie whose taste will remind you of your favorite apple crumble.

1. In a blender, combine the oats and walnuts. Process with 20 to 30 (one-second) pulses, until finely ground.
2. Add the apple juice, yogurt, apples, nutmeg, vanilla, and ice (if using), and blend until smooth, about 2 minutes, stopping the blender if needed to scrape down the sides so everything is fully incorporated.
3. Pour into two glasses and enjoy.

Substitute It! Replace the walnuts with 2 tablespoons of almond butter. Add the almond butter in step 2, after pulsing the oats.

PER SERVING Calories: 456; Total Fat: 13 g; Sugars: 56 g; Carbohydrates: 80 g; Fiber: 9 g; Protein: 9 g

Almond Butter, Banana, and Oatmeal Energy Blast

. . . .

Energy Boost

Kid Friendly

Makes 2 (10-ounce) servings
Prep time: 5 minutes

½ cup rolled oats

2 cups unsweetened nondairy or dairy milk of choice

2 tablespoons almond butter

1 frozen banana

¼ cup crushed ice (optional)

If any two flavors were born to go together, it's almond butter and banana. This hearty smoothie is an AB&B lover's dream. Additionally, the fat and protein in the almond butter allows you to have this smoothie for breakfast and not be starving 10 minutes later.

1. Put the oats in a blender. Process with 20 to 30 (one-second) pulses, until finely ground.
2. Add the milk, almond butter, banana, and ice (if using), and blend until smooth, about 2 minutes, stopping the blender if needed to scrape down the sides so everything is fully incorporated.
3. Pour into two glasses and enjoy.

Simplify It! Have leftover oatmeal you made for breakfast? It will keep in the refrigerator for up to 3 days, and you can add ¾ cup in place of the rolled oats. Then, you can skip the first step and just blend it all together.

PER SERVING Calories: 313; Total Fat: 17 g; Sugars: 8 g; Carbohydrates: 33 g; Fiber: 7 g; Protein: 8 g

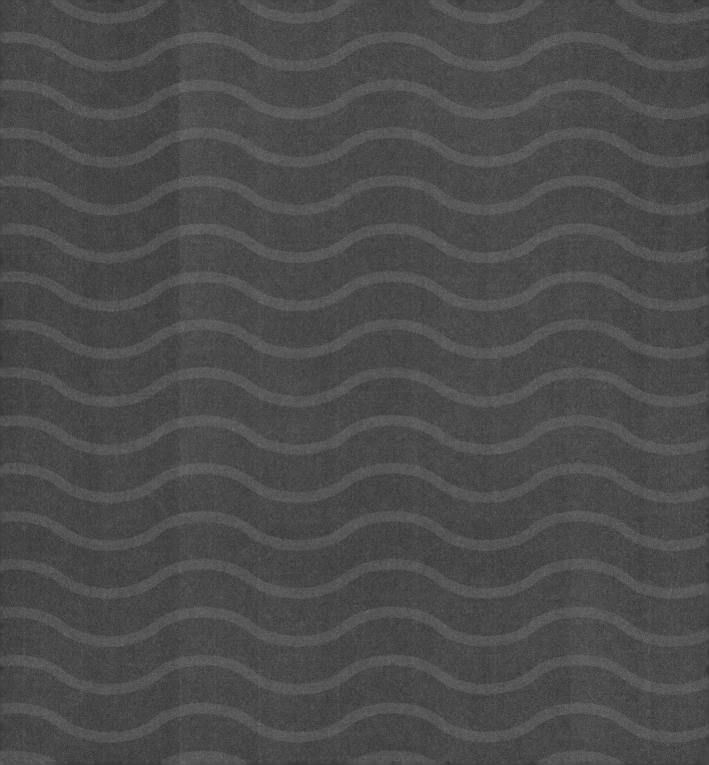

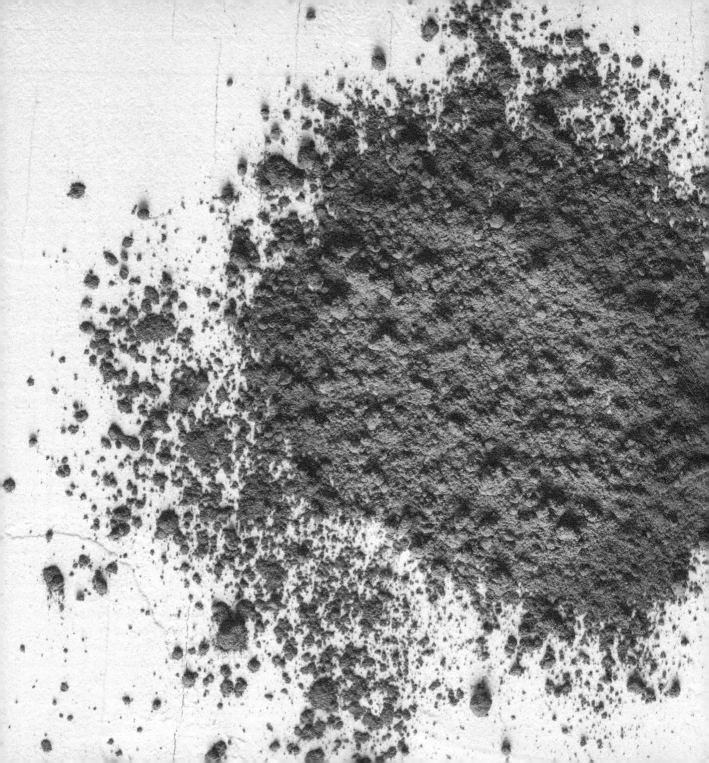

Part Two

Superfood Boosts

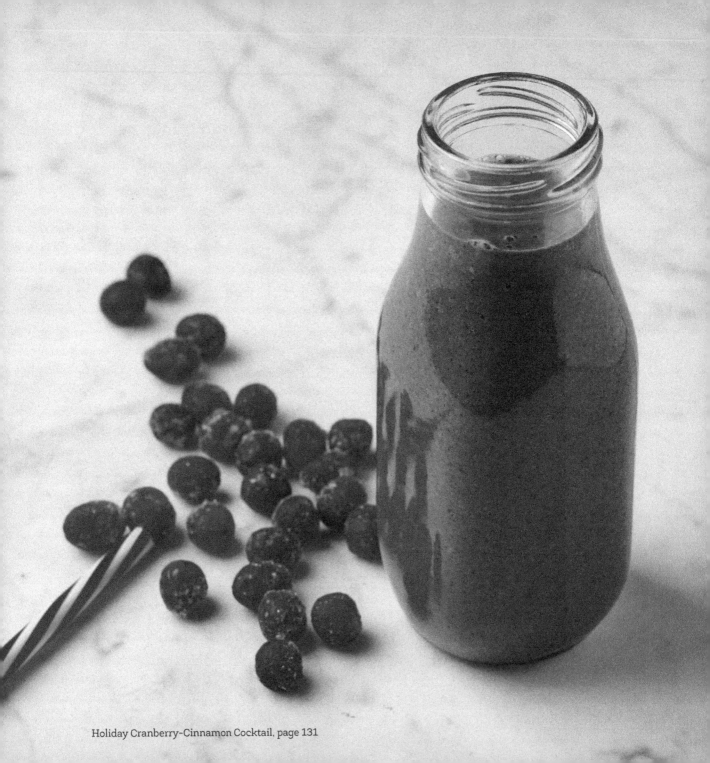

Holiday Cranberry-Cinnamon Cocktail, page 131

Chapter Nine

Cinnamon

Cinnamon has been well loved for centuries as both a culinary and medicinal spice. It's easy to adore cinnamon's sweet and slightly spicy taste, which adds depth and enhances flavors. More impressive are cinnamon's vast health benefits. It's rich in antioxidants and anti-inflammatory compounds that battle pain, boost the immune system, and inhibit cancer cells. But that is only the tip of the iceberg: Cinnamon helps lower blood sugar and cholesterol levels, freshens your breath, enhances memory and brain function, supports digestive health, and fights off bacteria, yeast, and fungus.

There are two common types of cinnamon: Ceylon, also called "true cinnamon," and Cassia. Ceylon is milder, sweeter, and of higher quality than Cassia, but it is also more expensive and sometimes trickier to find. Cassia has stronger and spicier flavor notes, is of lower quality and cheaper than Ceylon, and contains much higher levels of coumarin, a compound linked to liver and kidney damage when consumed in large doses. Because I like to use cinnamon a lot in smoothies, baking, and savory recipes, I prefer to purchase Ceylon cinnamon.

Common forms: Cinnamon sticks, ground, and essential oil; ground cinnamon is the best option for smoothies.

Where to find them: In the spice aisle at your local grocery or health food store or online.

Prep tip: If you have a good spice grinder or a high-speed blender, you can pulverize your own ground cinnamon from cinnamon sticks.

Sweet Cinnamon Bun Smoothie

Anti-Inflammatory

Energy Boost

Makes 2 (8-ounce) servings
Prep time: 5 minutes

1 cup water
½ cup plain, unsweetened nondairy or dairy yogurt or kefir of choice (store-bought or homemade, page 70)
¼ cup rolled oats
1 frozen banana
2 tablespoons almond butter or ground pecans
1 tablespoon ground cinnamon
½ teaspoon vanilla extract
Pinch salt
Pinch ground nutmeg (optional)

Swap your morning pastry with this sweet and simple cinnamon bun smoothie. It has all the flavor notes of a traditional cinnamon bun, with the added benefit of anti-inflammatory nutrients, protein, digestion-friendly probiotics, and fiber.

1. In a blender, combine the water, yogurt, oats, banana, almond butter, cinnamon, vanilla, salt, and nutmeg (if using). Blend until smooth, about 1 minute, stopping the blender if needed to scrape down the sides so everything is fully incorporated.
2. Pour into two glasses and enjoy.

Taste Tip: For extra creaminess, use 1 cup of full-fat coconut milk instead of water.

PER SERVING Calories: 246; Total Fat: 11 g; Sugars: 13 g; Carbohydrates: 31 g; Fiber: 5 g; Protein: 8 g

Cinnamon Cherry Pie Smoothie

Anti-Inflammatory
Heart Healthy

Makes 2 (10-ounce) servings
Prep time: 5 minutes

1½ cups water or nondairy or
  dairy milk of choice
1½ cups frozen, pitted cherries
⅓ cup cashews, soaked and
  drained, or 3 tablespoons
  cashew butter
1 tablespoon ground cinnamon
1 teaspoon freshly squeezed
  lemon juice
½ teaspoon vanilla extract
Pinch salt

Start your day off on a high note with cherries, which reduce inflammation and swelling in the joints and cardiovascular system and help improve your mood. If you'd like to make this a green smoothie, just add a cup of your favorite dark leafy greens.

1. In a blender, combine the water, cherries, cashews, cinnamon, lemon juice, vanilla, and salt. Blend until smooth, about 2 minutes, stopping the blender if needed to scrape down the sides so everything is fully incorporated.
2. Pour into two glasses and enjoy.

Substitute It! Swap the cherries for 2 cups of any berry to transform the flavor of this smoothie. Strawberries, blueberries, raspberries, and blackberries all work well. If you use cranberries, you'll need an additional sweetener, or mix half cranberries and half sweet berries.

PER SERVING Calories: 228; Total Fat: 12 g; Sugars: 17 g; Carbohydrates: 32 g; Fiber: 5 g; Protein: 5 g

Blueberry-Cinnamon Antioxidant Dynamo

Anti-Inflammatory

Greens Lover

Immunity Boost

Makes 2 (14-ounce) servings

Prep time: 5 minutes

1½ cups water or nondairy or
dairy milk of choice

¼ cup plain, unsweetened
nondairy or dairy yogurt or
kefir or choice (store-bought
or homemade, page 70)

2 cups frozen blueberries

1 cup spinach, tightly packed

¼ cup sunflower seed butter

1 tablespoon ground cinnamon

1 date, pitted

Antioxidant-rich blueberries, greens, and cinnamon combine to make this a powerhouse smoothie that contains plenty of natural sweetness. It's a delicious way to start the day and is sure to keep you energized and satisfied.

1. In a blender, combine the water, yogurt, blueberries, spinach, sunflower seed butter, cinnamon, and date. Blend until smooth, about 2 minutes, stopping the blender if needed to scrape down the sides so everything is fully incorporated.

2. Pour into two glasses and enjoy.

✳ **Power Up!** Spoon 1 to 2 tablespoons of chia seeds into the blender for more fiber, anti-inflammatory fats, and a thicker texture.

PER SERVING Calories: 314; Total Fat: 16 g; Sugars: 19 g; Carbohydrates: 38 g; Fiber: 6 g; Protein: 10 g

Morning Glory Muffin Smoothie

Energy Boost

Meal Swap

Makes 2 (16-ounce) servings

Prep time: 5 minutes

1¼ cups water or nondairy or
dairy milk of choice

1 cup grated carrots

2 apples, chopped into
1-inch chunks

½ cup frozen pineapple chunks

½ cup walnuts or pecans
(or ¼ cup nut butter of choice)

¼ cup unsweetened
shredded coconut

¼ cup rolled oats

1 tablespoon ground cinnamon

¼ teaspoon vanilla extract

Pinch salt

2 tablespoons raisins or cranberries, for topping (optional)

1 tablespoon chopped nuts
or seeds, such as walnuts,
almonds, or pecans, for topping
(optional)

Perhaps we should switch the name of this chapter to "Smoothies That Taste Like Baked Goods." Treats are a terrific inspiration for smoothie recipes, as we can replicate flavors while amping up the health benefits. I love this particular smoothie for its texture as much as for its taste.

1. In a blender, combine the water, carrots, apples, pineapple, walnuts, coconut, oats, cinnamon, vanilla, and salt. Blend until smooth, about 2 minutes, stopping the blender if needed to scrape down the sides so everything is fully incorporated.
2. Pour into two glasses, top with the dried fruit and/or nuts (if using), and enjoy.

Simplify It! If you aren't crazy about the additional texture created by the shredded coconut and rolled oats, leave them out, or swap with ½ cup full-fat coconut milk, coconut yogurt, or coconut kefir (store-bought or homemade, page 70).

PER SERVING Calories: 479; Total Fat: 25 g; Sugars: 30 g; Carbohydrates: 62 g; Fiber: 13 g; Protein: 9 g

Sweet Carob-Cinnamon Delight

Anti-Inflammatory
Heart Healthy

Makes 2 (8-ounce) servings
Prep time: 5 minutes

1 cup water
½ cup plain, unsweetened
   nondairy or dairy yogurt or
   kefir of choice (store-bought or
   homemade, page 70)
1 frozen banana
¼ cup almond butter
2 tablespoons carob powder
1 tablespoon ground cinnamon
Pinch salt

I am on a mission to inspire a worldwide fondness for carob powder. Often eclipsed by cacao powder, carob deserves its own chance to sparkle. It offers a different yet lovable flavor profile than chocolate: It's earthier and sweeter and has an equally impressive nutritional profile, with an array of antioxidants, minerals like iron and calcium, and fiber. And unlike chocolate, it's caffeine-free.

1. In a blender, combine the water, yogurt, banana, almond butter, carob powder, cinnamon, and salt. Blend until smooth, about 1 minute, stopping the blender if needed to scrape down the sides so everything is fully incorporated.
2. Pour into two glasses and enjoy.

Substitute It! If you're not convinced you like carob, you can swap in cacao powder instead. You'll just have to live with my disappointment.

PER SERVING Calories: 355; Total Fat: 20 g; Sugars: 20 g; Carbohydrates: 38 g; Fiber: 7 g; Protein: 10 g

Cinnamon-Fig-Tahini-Maple Slim-Down

Heart Healthy

Weight Loss

Makes 2 (8-ounce) servings
Prep time: 5 minutes

1 cup water or nondairy or dairy milk of choice

¼ cup plain, unsweetened nondairy or dairy yogurt or kefir of choice (store-bought or homemade, page 70)

6 fresh figs, halved (can also freeze for a thicker texture)

1 frozen banana

¼ cup tahini

1½ tablespoons maple syrup

1 tablespoon ground cinnamon

Tahini and maple syrup (or honey) complement each other particularly well. In this smoothie, figs join the fray to offer additional sweetness, minerals, and fiber for blood sugar balance, cardiovascular health, and weight loss.

1. In a blender, combine the water, yogurt, figs, banana, tahini, maple syrup, and cinnamon. Blend until smooth, about 1 minute, stopping the blender if needed to scrape down the sides so everything is fully incorporated.

2. Pour into two glasses and enjoy.

Substitute It! If you can't locate fresh figs, use about ⅓ cup of dried figs and soak them in warm water for 30 minutes to soften before blending. You can also save that water for future smoothies.

PER SERVING Calories: 411; Total Fat: 17 g; Sugars: 43 g; Carbohydrates: 64 g; Fiber: 11 g; Protein: 9 g

Holiday Cranberry-Cinnamon Cocktail

Anti-Inflammatory

Heart Healthy

Makes 2 (10-ounce) servings
Prep time: 5 minutes

1¼ cups cashew milk
½ cup fresh or frozen
     cranberries
½ cup frozen raspberries
1 orange, peeled and chopped
     into 1-inch chunks
¼ cup almond butter
1 tablespoon honey or
     maple syrup
1 tablespoon ground cinnamon
¼ teaspoon ground nutmeg
Pinch ground allspice
Pinch ground cloves

This gently spiced smoothie combines heart-healthy cranberries, oranges, and cinnamon to create a delicious cocktail you'll want to sip all year round. Who says you can't channel the holiday season every day of the year?

1. In a blender, combine the cashew milk, cranberries, raspberries, orange, almond butter, honey, cinnamon, nutmeg, allspice, and cloves. Blend until smooth, about 1 minute, stopping the blender if needed to scrape down the sides so everything is fully incorporated.
2. Pour into two glasses and enjoy.

✳ **Power Up!** Add 1 cup of spinach for an array of anti-inflammatory compounds, vitamins, and minerals, or 1 cup of kale if you can handle a little extra bitterness!

PER SERVING Calories: 326; Total Fat: 21 g; Sugars: 21 g; Carbohydrates: 35 g; Fiber: 8 g; Protein: 6 g

Heart-Healthy Apple-Cinnamon Smoothie

Anti-Inflammatory

Greens Lover

Heart Healthy

Kid Friendly

Makes 2 (12-ounce) servings
Prep time: 5 minutes

---

1 cup water or nondairy or dairy
    milk of choice

½ cup plain, unsweetened
    nondairy or dairy yogurt or
    kefir of choice (store-bought
    or homemade, page 70)

½ cup spinach, lightly packed

½ cup rolled oats

2 apples, chopped into 1-inch
    chunks (a sweeter variety
    works well: Fuji, Pink Lady,
    Red Delicious, Gala, etc.)

2 tablespoons almond butter

1 tablespoon ground cinnamon

Pinch ground nutmeg

Pinch ground cardamom

An apple pie in smoothie form, this beverage is packed to the brim with vitamins, minerals, and fiber that keep your heart healthy and strong, plus a touch of probiotics to keep your digestive system humming. While this smoothie is sweet on its own from the apples and spices, you can add one or two dates to make it extra kid-friendly.

1. In a blender, combine the water, yogurt, spinach, oats, apples, almond butter, cinnamon, nutmeg, and cardamom. Blend until smooth, about 1 minute, stopping the blender if needed to scrape down the sides so everything is fully incorporated.

2. Pour into two glasses and enjoy.

Simplify It! Not in the mood for a green smoothie? Ditch the spinach.

PER SERVING Calories: 347; Total Fat: 12 g; Sugars: 29 g; Carbohydrates: 55 g; Fiber: 10 g; Protein: 10 g

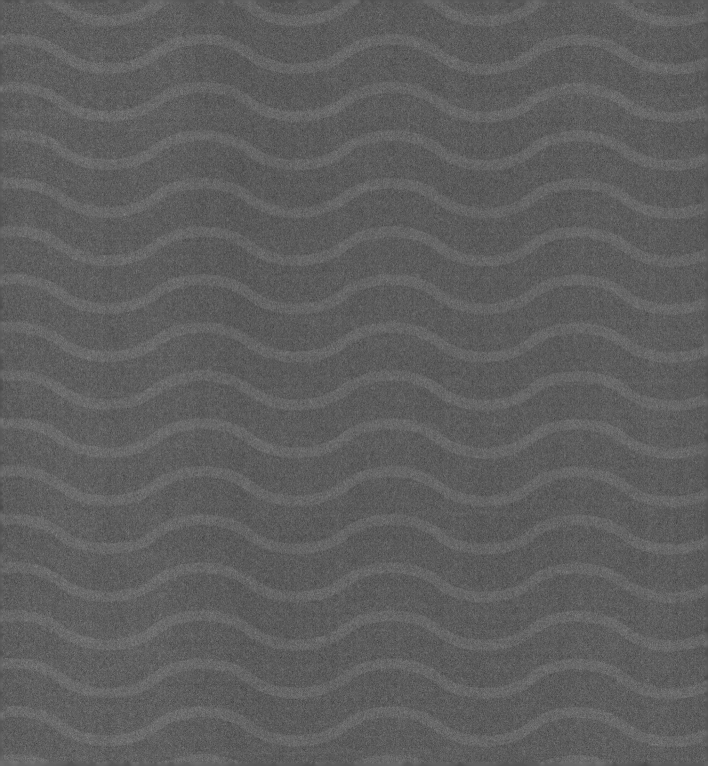

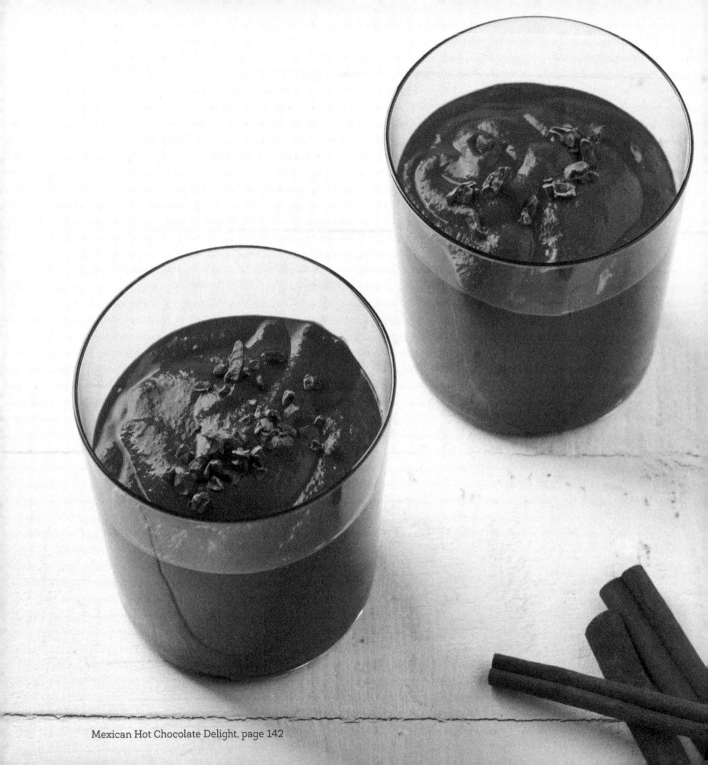

Mexican Hot Chocolate Delight, page 142

Chapter Ten

Cacao/Cocoa

I don't want to live in a world without chocolate.

Once highly prized by the Aztecs and even used as a form of currency, chocolate continues to be one of the most popular confections.

Cacao powder is extracted from the cocoa bean—a fruit—and then dried, while sweeter cocoa powder is roasted at a higher temperature. Cacao has a plethora of compounds that are beneficial to our health. It contains a payload of antioxidants—more than red wine, green tea, blueberries, and acai—that work to dampen inflammation. Cacao is especially beneficial to the digestive tract and the cardiovascular system, areas of the body susceptible to damage.

If you're interested in a mood boost, dark chocolate contains several compounds that may help. Anandamide attaches to the cannabinoid receptors in our brains, impersonating the effects of cannabis drugs, while phenylethylamine, also known as the "love chemical," floods our brains with dopamine and fills us with bliss. In addition, the compound theobromine possesses stimulant properties without the negative effects of caffeine.

And I'm not finished extolling chocolate's many wonders. It contains iron to support energy levels; magnesium for relaxation, strong bones, and cardiovascular function; and compounds that enhance immunity, inhibit the growth of cancer cells, and improve skin elasticity. Consumption of chocolate has even been shown to boost cognitive function and limit brain aging.

Chocolate quality is important: The darker the better, as it will contain much less sugar. Read labels to avoid preservatives and artificial colors and flavors. Cacao and cocoa powders are easy to blend into smoothies and should consist of just a single ingredient; but again, be sure to check the label.

I prefer cacao powder over cocoa powder in smoothies. While it can be the more bitter choice, depending on the bean's origin, it has a depth of flavor and robust quality that I prefer: In short, it just tastes more chocolaty!

Common forms: Cacao and cocoa powder, cacao butter (the pure fat), and cacao nibs (broken bits of the cacao bean). The powder is best for blending into smoothies, while the nibs can be sprinkled on top for flavor and crunch.

Where to find them: The baking aisle of your grocery store, online, or at a health food store.

Prep tip: If you are using a lot of cacao powder in a smoothie, you can add it after the liquids to ensure it is fully blended. Cacao is best stored in the pantry or another cool, dark place.

Chocolate-Cauliflower Milk Shake

Anti-Inflammatory Immunity Boost

Makes 2 (8-ounce) servings
Prep time: 5 minutes

1 cup nondairy or dairy milk
of choice
2 tablespoons cacao powder
¾ cup cauliflower florets, frozen
1 frozen banana
2 tablespoons almond butter

As I mentioned in chapter 3, cauliflower may seem like an odd smoothie ingredient. But it is startlingly mild, so you will barely realize it's there, while enjoying the anti-inflammatory, detoxifying, and anti-cancer benefits. Tossing raw cauliflower florets into the freezer is the easiest prep option, but you can also steam them first and then freeze if you're worried they will taste too "raw," or if you have a weak blender.

1. In a blender, combine the milk, cacao, cauliflower, banana, and almond butter. Blend until smooth, about 2 minutes, stopping the blender if needed to scrape down the sides so everything is fully incorporated.
2. Pour into two glasses and enjoy.

✶ **Power Up!** Add a teaspoon of ground cinnamon for more anti-inflammatory compounds and a slightly sweeter flavor.

PER SERVING Calories: 255; Total Fat: 17 g; Sugars: 9 g; Carbohydrates: 30 g; Fiber: 10 g; Protein: 9 g

Black Forest Antioxidant Smoothie

Anti-Inflammatory

Greens Lover

Heart Healthy

Meal Swap

Makes 2 (10-ounce) servings
Prep time: 5 minutes

---

1 cup nondairy or dairy milk
    of choice

½ cup nondairy or dairy kefir or
    yogurt of choice (store-bought
    or homemade, page 70)

¼ cup cacao powder

½ cup spinach, lightly packed

1 cup frozen cherries, pitted

1 frozen banana

¼ cup rolled oats

2 tablespoons chia seeds

Deeply rich and satisfying, this smoothie will make you forget about the cake version. It's chock-full of antioxidants from the cacao, cherries, spinach, and chia seeds, which will help protect the heart, skin, and immune system. For an extra touch of decadence, top this with a dollop of coconut whipped cream!

1. In a blender, combine the milk, yogurt, cacao, spinach, cherries, banana, oats, and chia seeds. Blend until smooth, about 2 minutes, stopping the blender if needed to scrape down the sides so everything is fully incorporated.
2. Pour into two glasses and enjoy.

Substitute It! Subbing in flaxseed will still provide protein, fiber, and fat—plus offer some hormone-balancing properties.

PER SERVING Calories: 382; Total Fat: 17 g; Sugars: 19 g; Carbohydrates: 61 g; Fiber: 22 g; Protein: 18 g

Blueberry-Cacao Double Indemnity

Anti-Inflammatory

Greens Lover

Immunity Boost

Meal Swap

Makes 2 (14-ounce) servings
Prep time: 5 minutes

1½ cups water or nondairy or
   dairy milk of choice
2 tablespoons cacao powder
1½ cups spinach, lightly packed
   (see tip)
1½ cups fresh or frozen
   blueberries
1 frozen banana
1 avocado, peeled and pitted
2 tablespoons almond butter

This is one of the first green smoothie recipes I ever created, so it holds a special place in my heart. Aside from being delicious, the blueberry-chocolate combo enhances the nutritional power of both foods! I prefer using cacao powder in this recipe for its full-bodied, chocolaty flavor. If you have cocoa powder on hand, you may want to start at 1 tablespoon and add more as needed.

1. In a blender, combine the water, cacao, spinach, blueberries, banana, avocado, and almond butter. Blend until smooth, about 2 minutes, stopping the blender if needed to scrape down the sides so everything is fully incorporated.
2. Pour into two glasses and enjoy.

Substitute It! This recipe also works well with kale instead of spinach.

PER SERVING Calories: 416; Total Fat: 28 g; Sugars: 19 g; Carbohydrates: 51 g; Fiber: 17 g; Protein: 10 g

Chocolate-Coconut Snowball Energy Surge

Energy Boost
Kid Friendly

Makes 2 (8-ounce) servings
Prep time: 5 minutes

1 cup cashew milk
½ cup plain, unsweetened, coconut yogurt or coconut kefir (store-bought or homemade, page 70)
3 tablespoons cacao powder
1 frozen banana
½ cup rolled oats
2 tablespoons flaxseed
2 tablespoons unsweetened shredded coconut

Creamy cashew milk and coconut yogurt help transform the popular cookie into smoothie form. You'll love the toothsome flavor and texture here, and the smoothie's fiber will keep your energy levels high!

1. In a blender, combine the cashew milk, yogurt, cacao, banana, oats, flaxseed, and coconut. Blend until smooth, about 1 minute, stopping the blender if needed to scrape down the sides so everything is fully incorporated.
2. Pour into two glasses and enjoy.

Taste Tip: For a fruity flair, add ½ cup of your favorite berries—strawberries are always a hit!

PER SERVING Calories: 358; Total Fat: 18 g; Sugars: 11 g; Carbohydrates: 52 g; Fiber: 17 g; Protein: 14 g

Mexican Hot Chocolate Delight

Anti-Inflammatory
Heart Healthy

Makes 2 (8-ounce) servings
Prep time: 5 minutes

1 cup water or nondairy or dairy
    milk of choice
1 cup cooked, mashed sweet
    potato (about 2 medium pota-
    toes—keep the skins on for
    extra nutrients)
¼ cup cacao powder
2 tablespoons sunflower seed
    butter or almond butter
1 tablespoon ground cinnamon
⅛ teaspoon ground cayenne
    pepper, or more/less to taste
Pinch salt

You might imagine a fiery spice like cayenne could only cause pain, but it's actually the opposite. Capsaicin, one of the main compounds in cayenne and other chiles, inhibits inflammatory processes and *relieves* pain—apply some the next time you cut your finger! It also lowers blood pressure, stimulates blood flow, clears congestion, and boosts immunity. I have a low tolerance for spicy food, so there is minimal cayenne in this recipe, but feel free to add as much as you can handle.

1. In a blender, combine the water, sweet potato, cacao, sunflower seed butter, cinnamon, cayenne, and salt. Blend until smooth, about 2 minutes, stopping the blender if needed to scrape down the sides so everything is fully incorporated.
2. Pour into two glasses and enjoy.

Prep Tip: Create a breakfast pudding by adding ¼ cup chia seeds and 2 tablespoons rolled oats. Let set overnight, then stir in the morning.

PER SERVING Calories: 330; Total Fat: 16 g; Sugars: 7 g; Carbohydrates: 57 g; Fiber: 16 g; Protein: 14 g

Nutrient-Packed Chocolate-Mint Indulgence

· ·

Greens Lover

Meal Swap

Makes 2 (8-ounce) servings
Prep time: 5 minutes

1¼ cups water or nondairy or
    dairy milk of choice
2 tablespoons cacao powder
1 cup spinach, tightly packed
10 fresh mint leaves, ½ teaspoon
    peppermint extract, or 2 to
    3 drops food-grade peppermint
    essential oil
1 frozen banana
¼ cup almond butter or
    ground almonds
1 date, pitted

There are few flavor pairings more delicious than chocolate and mint, and I simply don't understand those who don't love it as I do. This smoothie captures the essence of your favorite mint-chocolate confection, with a heck of a lot more nutrients, such as antioxidants, fiber, and digestion-friendly and anti-inflammatory compounds. If you don't have mint leaves, peppermint extract, or oil, try 1¼ cups chilled mint tea.

1. In a blender, combine the water, cacao, spinach, mint, banana, almond butter, and date. Blend until smooth, about 2 minutes, stopping the blender if needed to scrape down the sides so everything is fully incorporated.
2. Pour into two glasses and enjoy.

✳ **Power Up!** Drop in ⅓ cup plain, unsweetened nondairy or dairy yogurt or kefir of your choice (store-bought or home-made, page 70) for digestion-supportive probiotics and additional fat, which lends more creaminess.

PER SERVING Calories: 320; Total Fat: 23 g; Sugars: 12 g; Carbohydrates: 34 g; Fiber: 9 g; Protein: 10 g

Chocolate-Raspberry Tart Smoothie

Greens Lover

Heart Healthy

Meal Swap

Weight Loss

Makes 2 (14-ounce) servings
Prep time: 5 minutes

1½ cups water or nondairy or
  dairy milk of choice

2 tablespoons cacao powder

1 cup spinach or kale, lightly
  packed (see tip)

2½ cups frozen raspberries
  (see headnote)

¼ cup sunflower seed butter,
  tahini, or almond butter

2 dates

½ teaspoon ground cinnamon

The combination of raspberries and chocolate has a fruity, sweet-and-tart mix of flavors, along with a boost of antioxidants. If you don't have raspberries on hand, blueberries or strawberries are a great substitute but sweeter, so you can probably skip the dates.

1. In a blender, combine the water, cacao, kale, raspberries, sunflower seed butter, dates, and cinnamon. Blend until smooth, about 2 minutes, stopping the blender if needed to scrape down the sides so everything is fully incorporated.
2. Pour into two glasses and enjoy.

Simplify It! Skip the greens for a brighter smoothie color and easier prep.

PER SERVING Calories: 344; Total Fat: 20 g; Sugars: 12 g; Carbohydrates: 44 g; Fiber: 17 g; Protein: 13 g

Mocha-Almond Energizer

Energy Boost

Makes 2 (8-ounce) servings
Prep time: 5 minutes

1 cup almond milk
½ cup chilled coffee, or herbal
   coffee alternative
½ cup plain, unsweetened nondairy or dairy yogurt or kefir of
   choice (store-bought or homemade, page 70)
3 tablespoons cacao powder
1 frozen banana
2 tablespoons flaxseed
2 tablespoons chopped almonds
   (toasted for extra flavor,
   see Prep Tip)

Coffee and chocolate are a popular combo, and in this smoothie, both flavors meld in perfect harmony without overpowering one another. As a side note, if you freeze this recipe in popsicle molds, it'll make a lovely summer treat!

1. In a blender, combine the almond milk, coffee, yogurt, cacao, banana, and flaxseed. Blend until smooth, about 1 minute, stopping the blender if needed to scrape down the sides so everything is fully incorporated.
2. Stir the almonds in by hand, pour into two glasses, and enjoy.

Taste Tip: If this smoothie isn't sweet enough, stir in some maple syrup or honey. You can also add crushed ice for a frostier texture.

Prep Tip: To toast almonds, preheat the oven to 350°F. Spread them on a baking sheet in an even layer and bake for 7 to 10 minutes, until lightly golden brown. Stir halfway through toasting to ensure even browning, and check frequently near the end to avoid burning.

PER SERVING Calories: 317; Total Fat: 17 g; Sugars: 12 g; Carbohydrates: 40 g; Fiber: 16 g; Protein: 16 g

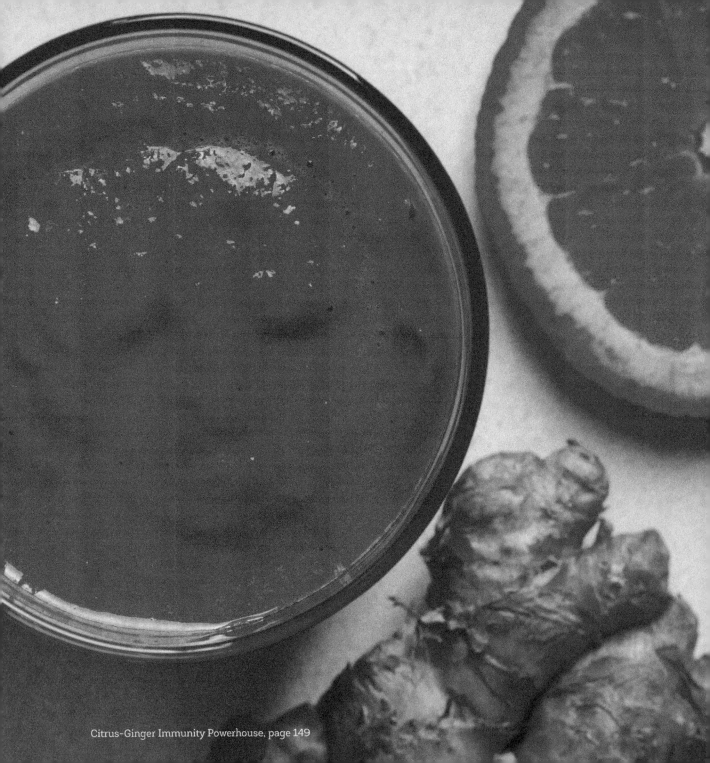

Citrus-Ginger Immunity Powerhouse, page 149

Chapter Eleven

Ginger

It can take some time to adapt to the spicy, pungent flavor of ginger, but it's well worth making the effort. Much of ginger's health benefits stem from compounds called gingerols, which block inflammation and can reduce both acute and chronic pain. They also have anti-cancer actions and enhance the immune system.

Ginger is renowned as a digestive aid, relieving motion sickness and nausea, and improving the symptoms of a range of gastrointestinal conditions. It also functions as an excellent carminative (which helps us relieve gas).

As I mentioned in the previous chapter, I have a low tolerance for spicy foods, so it took me some time to adjust to ginger, even though I wanted to love it right away because of its health benefits. I began with about ¼ teaspoon of fresh ginger in smoothies, and by now I've graduated to a full teaspoon.

Common forms: Fresh and dried.

Where to find them: Fresh ginger will be in the produce section of your grocery store, and dried in the spice aisle.

Prep tip: You don't need to peel ginger, but if you prefer it peeled, the best method is to scrape the peel off with a small spoon. This mainly removes the thin skin without too much of what's beneath.

Citrus-Ginger Immunity Powerhouse

Anti-Inflammatory

Greens Lover

Immunity Boost

Makes 2 (12-ounce) servings
Prep time: 5 minutes

¾ **cup water**

¾ **cup freshly squeezed orange juice (about 3 oranges)**

2 **cups spinach, lightly packed**

2 **pears, chopped into 1-inch chunks**

1 **avocado**

1½ **teaspoons grated fresh ginger or ¾ teaspoon ground (or more/less to taste)**

Handful crushed ice

Give colds and flus a run for their money with this powerful smoothie! Packed with vitamin C and anti-inflammatory, immune-boosting ginger compounds, this smoothie has the added benefit of pears, a fruit rich in fiber and antioxidants that decrease our risk of disease.

1. In a blender, combine the water, orange juice, spinach, pears, avocado, ginger, and ice. Blend until smooth, about 2 minutes, stopping the blender if needed to scrape down the sides so everything is fully incorporated.
2. Pour into two glasses and enjoy.

Substitute It! For a spicier kick, substitute half of the spinach with arugula or watercress.

PER SERVING Calories: 316; Total Fat: 14 g; Sugars: 29 g; Carbohydrates: 50 g; Fiber: 13 g; Protein: 4 g

Strawberry-Ginger Anti-Inflammatory Boost

Anti-Inflammatory

Greens Lover

Kid Friendly

Makes 2 (14-ounce) servings
Prep time: 5 minutes

1½ cups water or nondairy or
    dairy milk of choice

2 cups spinach, lightly packed, or
    a half head of romaine lettuce

2 cups frozen strawberries,
    thawed 5 to 10 minutes for
    easier blending

½ cup plain, unsweetened
    nondairy or dairy yogurt or
    kefir of choice (store-bought or
    homemade, page 70)

¼ cup sunflower seed butter or
    almond butter

1 teaspoon grated fresh ginger or
    ½ teaspoon ground (or more/
    less to taste, see tip)

1 teaspoon ground cinnamon

This smoothie is a great introduction to ginger, as the berries, greens, and cinnamon all camouflage its spicy notes. For more luxury, use coconut milk instead of water (or half coconut milk, half water)—this helps temper the ginger, too.

1. In a blender, combine the water, spinach, strawberries, yogurt, sunflower seed butter, ginger, and cinnamon. Blend until smooth, about 2 minutes, stopping the blender if needed to scrape down the sides so everything is fully incorporated.

2. Pour into two glasses and enjoy.

✳ **Power Up!** Double the ginger to enhance its benefits and flavor, or throw in ½ teaspoon ground turmeric for additional anti-inflammatory properties.

PER SERVING Calories: 307; Total Fat: 20 g; Sugars: 6 g; Carbohydrates: 27 g; Fiber: 6 g; Protein: 9 g

Gingerbread Fuel Rush

Energy Boost
Kid Friendly

Makes 2 (10-ounce) servings
Prep time: 5 minutes

1 cup water or nondairy or dairy
   milk of choice
½ cup pumpkin purée
   (homemade or canned)
¼ cup plain, unsweetened
   nondairy or dairy yogurt or
   kefir of choice (store-bought or
   homemade, page 70)
2 tablespoons blackstrap
   molasses
1 frozen banana
¼ cup almond butter or
   2 tablespoons pecans
1 tablespoon ground cinnamon
1 teaspoon grated fresh ginger or
   ½ teaspoon ground (or more/
   less to taste)
⅛ teaspoon ground nutmeg
   (see tip)
⅛ teaspoon ground allspice
   (see tip)
Pinch ground cloves (see tip)
Pinch salt

This smoothie is sweetly spiced and full of flavor. You'll enjoy extra depth and nutrient richness from the pumpkin purée and blackstrap molasses. Molasses is a by-product from sugar manufacturing, but unlike refined sugar, it contains a wealth of nutrients like iron for energy, calcium and magnesium for bone health, and potassium for the heart. If you can't find blackstrap, another variety will suffice.

1. In a blender, combine the water, pumpkin purée, yogurt, molasses, banana, almond butter, cinnamon, ginger, nutmeg, allspice, cloves, and salt. Blend until smooth, about 1 minute, stopping the blender if needed to scrape down the sides so everything is fully incorporated.
2. Pour into two glasses and enjoy.

Simplify It! If you don't have spices like nutmeg, allspice, or cloves on hand, leave them out. The cinnamon and ginger will uphold the gingerbread vibe.

PER SERVING Calories: 364; Total Fat: 21 g; Sugars: 24 g; Carbohydrates: 45 g; Fiber: 7 g; Protein: 7 g

Squash, Maple, and Ginger Immunity Reboot

. . . .

Anti-Inflammatory Meal Swap

Makes 2 (12-ounce) servings
Prep time: 5 minutes

---

1 cup nondairy or dairy milk of choice
½ cup water
2 cups cubed butternut squash, steamed then frozen (see tip)
¼ cup tahini
2 tablespoons maple syrup
1½ teaspoons grated fresh ginger or ¾ teaspoon ground (or more/less to taste)
1 teaspoon ground cinnamon
Pinch salt

Butternut squash is not a common smoothie ingredient, but it's so darn nutritious, it should be! Winter squashes contain anti-inflammatory and immune-boosting compounds called cucurbitacins, along with fiber, antioxidant vitamins A and C, and even some beneficial omega-3 fatty acids. I adore this combination of flavors and hope you will, too!

1. In a blender, combine the milk, water, squash, tahini, maple syrup, ginger, cinnamon, and salt. Blend until smooth, about 2 minutes, stopping the blender if needed to scrape down the sides so everything is fully incorporated.
2. Pour into two glasses and enjoy.

Prep Tip: Steam and freeze the squash in advance. I have tried this recipe with both steamed/frozen cubes and purée, and I much prefer the texture of the former. However, if you have small ice cube trays, you can freeze the purée and use 1½ cups of cubes.

PER SERVING Calories: 360; Total Fat: 19 g; Sugars: 16 g; Carbohydrates: 44 g; Fiber: 11 g; Protein: 8 g

Ginger, Lemon, and Kale Vitality Lift

Greens Lover

Immunity Boost

Makes 2 (14-ounce) servings
Prep time: 5 minutes

1½ cups water
2 curly kale leaves, stemmed and
  torn into pieces (about 2 cups)
1 cup frozen pineapple chunks
1 green apple, cored and cut into
  1-inch chunks
¼ cup hemp seeds
2 tablespoons freshly squeezed
  lemon juice
1½ teaspoons grated fresh ginger
  or ¾ teaspoon ground (or more/
  less to taste)

Bitter, sour, spicy, and sweet flavors combine in this fantastic green smoothie. You're experiencing almost all five tastes in one glass! Aside from the flavor, you can rest assured that your immune system is well taken care of with a surfeit of vitamins C and A as well as iron.

1. In a blender, combine the water, kale, pineapple, apple, hemp seeds, lemon juice, and ginger. Blend until smooth, about 2 minutes, stopping the blender if needed to scrape down the sides so everything is fully incorporated.
2. Pour into two glasses and enjoy.

Taste Tip: If you need more sweetness in this smoothie, add half a frozen banana.

PER SERVING Calories: 258; Total Fat: 6 g; Sugars: 20 g; Carbohydrates: 34 g; Fiber: 5 g; Protein: 6 g

Beet-Ginger Detox

Anti-Inflammatory

Energy Boost

Weight Loss

Makes 2 (12-ounce) servings

Prep time: 5 minutes

---

1 cup water or nondairy or dairy
   milk of choice

1 cup grated beets

1 cup frozen raspberries

1 orange, peeled and chopped into
   1-inch chunks

1 (4-inch) piece cucumber,
   chopped into 1-inch chunks

2 tablespoons ground flaxseed

1½ teaspoons grated fresh ginger
   or ¾ teaspoon ground ginger
   (or more/less to taste)

Zest and juice of 1 lime

I'm not a fan of extreme detox diets; instead, I feel it's gentler to aid your body's natural detoxification processes by adding specific foods to your diet that assist in different ways. Here, the betalains from the beets and the vitamin C from the lemon and cucumber help the liver filter out toxins. Meanwhile ginger stimulates digestion, and the fiber in the raspberries and flax ensures that we eliminate any unwanted chemicals.

1. In a blender, combine the water, beets, raspberries, orange, cucumber, flaxseed, ginger, and lime juice. Blend until smooth, about 2 minutes, stopping the blender if needed to scrape down the sides so everything is fully incorporated.
2. Pour into two glasses and enjoy.

✳ **Power Up!** Add ¼ cup pomegranate arils or ½ teaspoon ground turmeric for extra antioxidants and anti-inflammatory properties.

PER SERVING Calories: 185; Total Fat: 5 g; Sugars: 19 g; Carbohydrates: 33 g; Fiber: 11 g; Protein: 6 g

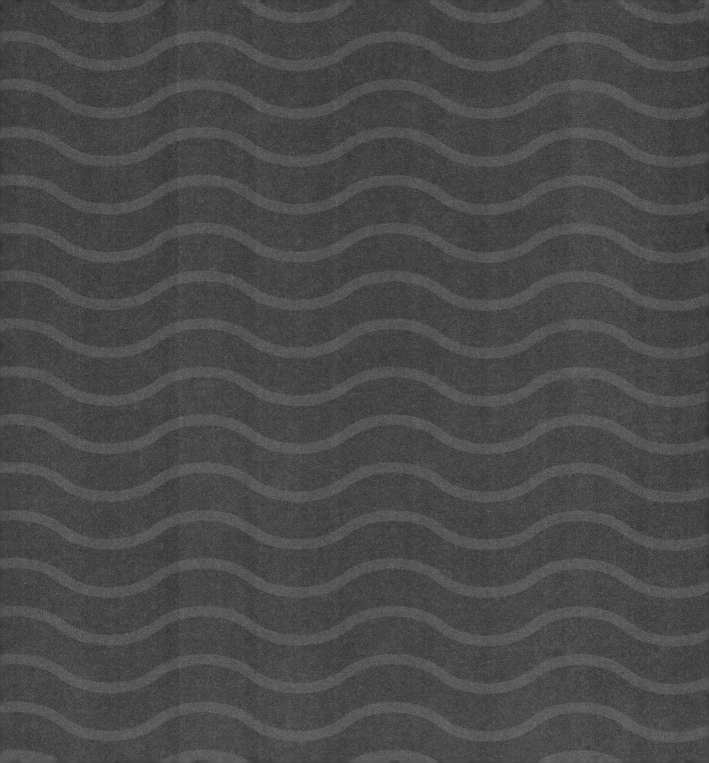

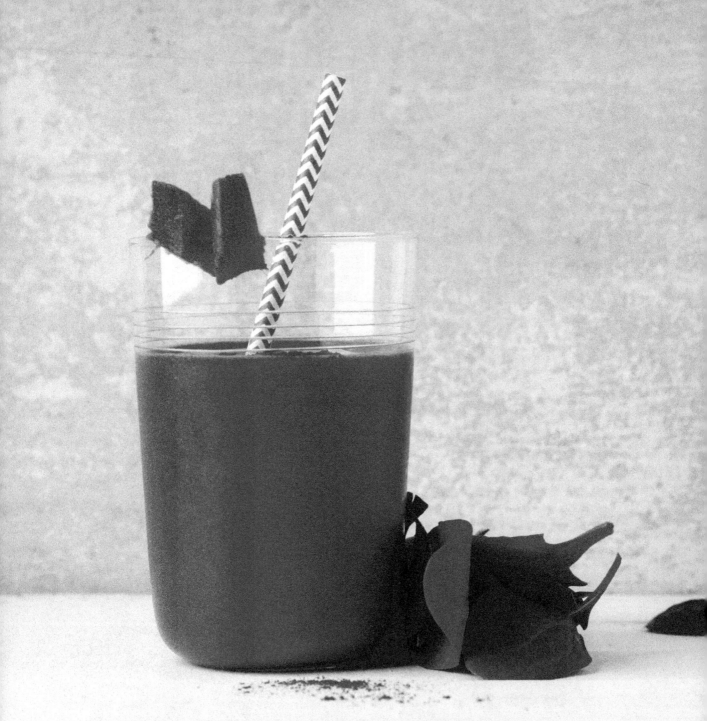

Mango-Turmeric Green Smoothie, page 162

Chapter Twelve

Turmeric

The long-standing adage "What's old is new again" is especially true with turmeric. It's been around for nearly 4,000 years, originating in India as a key spice in the Ayurvedic tradition of healing.

There are more than 100 constituents in turmeric, but the primary compound that lends turmeric its strength is called curcumin (it's also one of the most well-researched).

Curcumin has antioxidant properties and is extremely anti-inflammatory, inhibiting the processes that lead to inflammation. It has been shown to benefit multiple forms of arthritis, inflammatory bowel diseases, heart disease, cancers, obesity, and respiratory conditions.

But you don't have to be grappling with inflammation to consume it. Turmeric can help protect vital organs like the liver, brain, and heart from damage and decline and may prevent inflammation from occurring in the first place.

Turmeric root is related to ginger and has a bright orange-yellow hue and a bitter, spicy flavor.

Some people find turmeric more difficult to adapt to than ginger, so it's best to start really slow (⅛ teaspoon)—otherwise, you may find your smoothie unpalatable. Even if you like it, as I mentioned in the section "Using and Mixing Superfoods" (see page xix), adding several teaspoons to the blender will be so overpowering, it will ruin your smoothie.

You don't need to consume very much of this special spice to receive its benefits!

Common forms: Fresh and ground; both can work in smoothies, but ground is more widely available and is not as strongly flavored as fresh.

Where to find them: Ground turmeric will be in the spice aisle at your grocery store; fresh turmeric—if accessible—will likely be in the produce department.

Prep tip: Turmeric stains everything, from your hands to your blender to counters to tea towels. So take care when using it, especially if you are chopping or grating the fresh root. Not surprisingly, there are many home remedies to handle turmeric stains, including scrubbing with vinegar or lemon or applying a baking soda paste. Some also swear by leaving their turmeric-stained blender or clothing out in the sun.

"Golden Milk" Turmeric Smoothie

Anti-Inflammatory

Makes 2 (8-ounce) servings
Prep time: 5 minutes

1 cup full-fat coconut milk
1 frozen banana
½ cup sweet potato purée
  (or pumpkin)
1 tablespoon maple syrup, or
  more if desired
1 teaspoon ground turmeric
1 teaspoon ground cinnamon
1 teaspoon grated fresh ginger or
  ½ teaspoon ground ginger
¼ cup hemp seeds or
  2 tablespoons nut butter
  of choice

Golden milk, a hot turmeric tea or latte, is a popular beverage that has swept the health food world. You can easily enjoy it in smoothie form as well! I highly recommend using coconut milk instead of another nondairy milk, since not only does it make this drink super creamy but also because the fat content in coconut milk helps you better absorb turmeric's nutrients.

1. In a blender, combine the coconut milk, banana, sweet potato, maple syrup, turmeric, cinnamon, ginger, and hemp seeds. Blend until smooth, about 1 minute, stopping the blender if needed to scrape down the sides so everything is fully incorporated.
2. Pour into two glasses and enjoy.

✳ **Power Up!** For added "zing" and digestive benefits, try swapping half or all of the coconut milk for coconut kefir.

PER SERVING Calories: 528; Total Fat: 34 g; Sugars: 21 g; Carbohydrates: 39 g; Fiber: 7 g; Protein: 8 g

Hidden Turmeric and Mixed Berry Blend

Anti-Inflammatory

Greens Lover

Meal Swap

Makes 2 (14-ounce) servings

Prep time: 5 minutes

1½ cups water or nondairy or
   dairy milk of choice

1 cup spinach, lightly packed

1 cup frozen blueberries

1 cup frozen strawberries, thawed
   5 to 10 minutes for easier
   blending

¼ cup rolled oats

2 tablespoons sunflower seed
   butter, almond butter, or tahini

1 teaspoon ground turmeric

1 teaspoon ground cinnamon

Berries are the kind of ingredient that cooperates well with other ingredients, and turmeric is no exception. They make a wonderful foil for turmeric, and considering the busy traffic of flavors in this smoothie, you'll barely notice the turmeric is there.

1. In a blender, combine the water, spinach, blueberries, strawberries, oats, sunflower seed butter, turmeric, and cinnamon. Blend until smooth, about 2 minutes, stopping the blender if needed to scrape down the sides so everything is fully incorporated.

2. Pour into two glasses and enjoy.

Substitute It! You can use any berry in this recipe, or swap half a cup of berries for pomegranate arils or cherries.

PER SERVING Calories: 205; Total Fat: 9 g; Sugars: 11 g; Carbohydrates: 29 g; Fiber: 5 g; Protein: 6 g

Mango-Turmeric Green Smoothie

Anti-Inflammatory

Greens Lover

Makes 2 (14-ounce) servings
Prep time: 5 minutes

1½ cups water or nondairy or
   dairy milk of choice
½ cup plain, unsweetened
   nondairy or dairy yogurt or
   kefir of choice (store-bought or
   homemade, page 70)
2 cups spinach, lightly packed
   (see tip)
2 cups frozen mango
2 tablespoons ground almonds
1 teaspoon ground turmeric

Frozen or fresh mango is lovely, but it is also quite sweet.
Even though this recipe only calls for a small amount of turmeric, it's enough to provide some balance to that sweetness.

1. In a blender, combine the water, yogurt, spinach, mango,
   almonds, and turmeric. Blend until smooth, about
   2 minutes, stopping the blender if needed to scrape down
   the sides so everything is fully incorporated.
2. Pour into two glasses and enjoy.

Simplify It! If you're not in the mood for a green smoothie,
leave the spinach out. Just be aware that you'll end up with
smaller servings.

PER SERVING Calories: 182; Total Fat: 6 g; Sugars: 26 g;
Carbohydrates: 31 g; Fiber: 4 g; Protein: 6 g

Pineapple-Turmeric-Ginger Antioxidant Boost

Anti-Inflammatory

Greens Lover

Immunity Boost

Makes 2 (14-ounce) servings
Prep time: 5 minutes

1½ cups water or nondairy or
   dairy milk of choice
2 cups spinach, lightly packed
   (see tip)
2 cups frozen pineapple chunks
1 tablespoon freshly squeezed
   lemon juice
1 teaspoon ground turmeric
1 teaspoon grated fresh ginger or
   ½ teaspoon ground

Love your liver with this tropical smoothie: It contains not only liver-supportive turmeric but also ample amounts of antioxidants in form of lemon, spinach, and pineapple, which will help keep our livers chugging along. Our liver performs more than 500 tasks, so let's be sure to take care of it!

1. In a blender, combine the water, spinach, pineapple, lemon juice, turmeric, and ginger. Blend until smooth, about 2 minutes, stopping the blender if needed to scrape down the sides so everything is fully incorporated.
2. Pour into two glasses and enjoy.

Substitute It! Swapping the spinach for kale, chard, or collards will create a more bitter flavor.

PER SERVING Calories: 96; Total Fat: 1 g; Sugars: 16 g; Carbohydrates: 24 g; Fiber: 3 g; Protein: 2 g

Orange-Turmeric Anti-Aging Tonic

Anti-Aging

Anti-Inflammatory

Immunity Boost

Makes 2 (10-ounce) servings
Prep time: 5 minutes

1 cup nondairy or dairy milk
   of choice
2 small oranges, peeled and
   chopped into 1-inch chunks
1 frozen banana
1 teaspoon ground turmeric
½ teaspoon grated fresh ginger or
   ¼ teaspoon ground
¼ cup hemp seeds

Another golden smoothie, this beverage has a delightful mix of sweet, tangy, and spicy flavors. I've already mentioned in earlier chapters that vitamin C helps keep your skin supple and strong, but turmeric also assists: Its anti-inflammatory actions strengthen skin health and can slow down aging of the body and brain.

1. In a blender, combine the milk, oranges, banana, turmeric, ginger, and hemp seeds. Blend until smooth, about 1 minute, stopping the blender if needed to scrape down the sides so everything is fully incorporated.
2. Pour into two glasses and enjoy.

Substitute It! For additional vitamin C, swap the banana with ½ cup mango or pineapple.

PER SERVING Calories: 306; Total Fat: 5 g; Sugars: 25 g; Carbohydrates: 37 g; Fiber: 7 g; Protein: 7 g

Pumpkin Pie Smoothie, the Redux

Energy Boost

Meal Swap

Makes 2 (12-ounce) servings
Prep time: 5 minutes

---

1 cup full-fat coconut milk
1 cup pumpkin purée
    (homemade or canned)
½ cup plain, unsweetened
    nondairy or dairy kefir or
    yogurt of choice (store-bought
    or homemade, page 70)
½ cup rolled oats
1 frozen banana
1 tablespoon maple syrup
1 tablespoon ground cinnamon
1 teaspoon grated fresh ginger or
    ½ teaspoon ground
½ teaspoon ground turmeric
⅛ teaspoon ground nutmeg
Pinch ground allspice
Pinch ground cloves
Pinch salt

This recipe builds upon the version in chapter 2 (see page 23). This variation not only has more spices and nuance but also includes several additional power foods like kefir and oats. It's nice to have options: You can throw together version one when you're in a rush, then move on to this one when you have a little more time to prep.

1. In a blender, combine the coconut milk, pumpkin, kefir, oats, banana, maple syrup, cinnamon, ginger, turmeric, nutmeg, allspice, cloves, and salt. Blend until smooth, about 1 minute, stopping the blender if needed to scrape down the sides so everything is fully incorporated.
2. Pour into two glasses and enjoy.

✳ **Power Up!** This smoothie also tastes delicious with 2 tablespoons of cacao powder, which bumps up the antioxidant quotient.

PER SERVING Calories: 525; Total Fat: 33 g; Sugars: 24 g; Carbohydrates: 57 g; Fiber: 12 g; Protein: 10 g

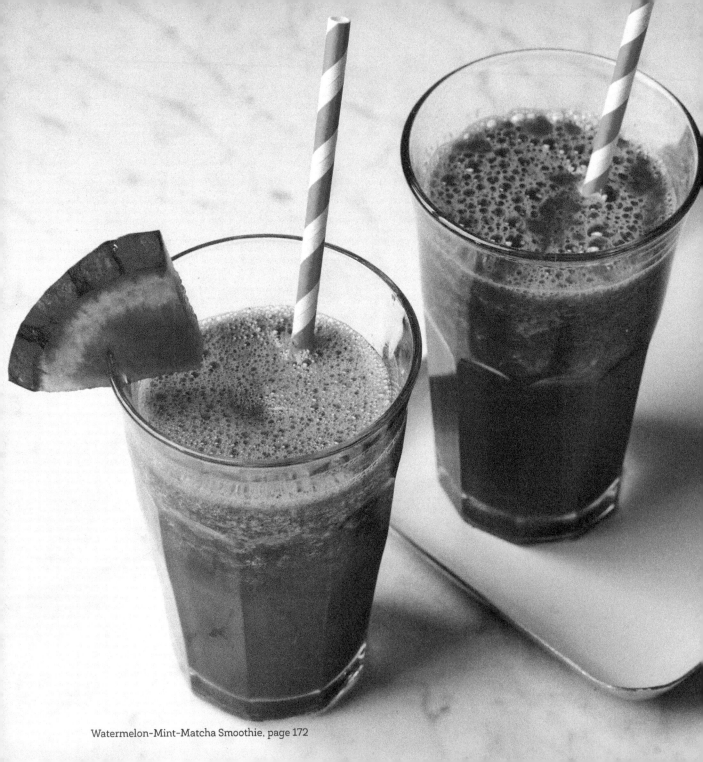

Watermelon-Mint-Matcha Smoothie, page 172

Chapter Thirteen

Green Tea and Matcha

ove tea? So do I! Tea isn't only for sipping. You can also chill it as a base for smoothies or throw a green tea powder like matcha into the mix.

Green tea and matcha come from the same plant but are grown and harvested differently. Matcha is kept in the shade, then the whole leaves are ground into a fine powder. It has a bright green color and a sweeter taste than green tea leaves, which are grown in sunlight and dried into loose-leaf tea.

Both green tea and matcha contain the antioxidant epigallocatechin gallate (EGCG), which lifts the immune system, reduces the risk of cancer and heart diseases, improves memory and cognition, thwarts inflammation, increases fat burn, and encourages weight loss. They also contain l-theanine, an amino acid that keeps us alert and focused yet relaxed, all at the same time.

Since you are consuming the entire leaf with matcha, rather than only steeping the leaves, matcha is much higher in antioxidants, amino acids, and caffeine. Yet both matcha and green tea are excellent choices for smoothies!

Common forms: Dried green tea leaves, culinary matcha, and ceremonial grade matcha. The latter is the most expensive.

Where to find them: Find green tea in the tea aisle of your grocery store or online. Matcha can be purchased at a health food store or online. If you have a specialty tea shop in your area, you may find both of these teas there.

Prep tip: Don't steep green tea leaves too long before chilling—a minute or two is all you need. This prevents bitterness in your smoothie.

Strawberry Green Tea Slim-Down

....

Anti-Inflammatory

Energy Boost

Weight Loss

Makes 2 (10-ounce) servings

Prep time: 5 minutes

**2 cups strongly brewed green
tea or jasmine green tea,
chilled (see tip)**

**3 cups fresh or frozen strawber-
ries, hulled and sliced**

**1 tablespoon grated fresh ginger
or 1 teaspoon ground**

¼ cup crushed ice (optional)

This simple smoothie is perfection with just a few ingredients. It features strawberries, which add sweetness to the
tannic flavor of green tea. This smoothie is full of antioxidants and vitamin C, and it also contains EGCG, a component
of green tea shown to be promising for weight loss.

1. In a blender, combine the tea, strawberries, ginger, and ice
   (if using). Blend until smooth, about 2 minutes, stopping
   the blender if needed to scrape down the sides so everything is fully incorporated.
2. Pour into two glasses and enjoy.

Taste Tip: For a stronger green tea flavor, freeze green tea in
ice cube trays and use it in place of the crushed ice.

PER SERVING Calories: 72; Total Fat: 1 g; Sugars: 11 g;
Carbohydrates: 17 g; Fiber: 4 g; Protein: 2 g

Green Melon Chai

**Anti-Inflammatory
Immunity Boost**

Makes 2 (12-ounce) servings
Prep time: 5 minutes

---

2 cups strong brew chai-flavored
  green tea, chilled (2 bags per
  8 ounces of water steeped for
  5 minutes)
2 cups cubed or balled fresh
  or frozen honeydew melon
  (see tip)
2 teaspoons grated fresh ginger
  or 1 teaspoon ground
½ teaspoon ground cinnamon
½ cup plain, unsweetened nondairy or dairy yogurt or kefir of
  choice (store-bought or homemade, page 70)

For this smoothie, you'll need chai-flavored green tea bags
to create a strong brew. The refreshing flavor of the melon
perfectly complements the delicate green tea flavor and chai
spices for an anti-inflammatory, energy-boosting tea.

1. In a blender, combine the tea, melon, ginger, cinnamon,
   and yogurt. Blend until smooth, about 2 minutes, stopping
   the blender if needed to scrape down the sides so everything is fully incorporated.
2. Pour into two glasses and enjoy.

Simplify It! Use frozen melon balls or purchase pre-
made, mixed melon balls from the produce section at the
grocery store.

PER SERVING Calories: 103; Total Fat: 2 g; Sugars: 17 g;
Carbohydrates: 19 g; Fiber: 2 g; Protein: 3 g

Tropical Mango-Matcha Escape

Energy Boost

Immunity Boost

Makes 2 (10-ounce) servings
Prep time: 5 minutes

2 cups unsweetened
   coconut water
1 cup chopped fresh or frozen
   unsweetened pineapple
1 cup chopped fresh or frozen
   mango (see tip)
¼ cup full-fat coconut milk
1 teaspoon matcha powder

Even if you can't get to an actual beach, this smoothie tastes like a seaside getaway. With pineapple, coconut, and mango, all you need to complete that vacation feel is an umbrella in your drink. It's also loaded with enzymes from the pineapple and antioxidants.

1. In a blender, combine the coconut water, pineapple, mango, coconut milk, and matcha powder. Blend until smooth, about 2 minutes, stopping the blender if needed to scrape down the sides so everything is fully incorporated.
2. Pour into two glasses and enjoy.

Prep Tip: To chop a mango, peel it with a vegetable peeler. Then, cut around the longest edge with a sharp paring knife. Twist the mango in half and remove the pit. Chop into cubes.

PER SERVING Calories: 233; Total Fat: 9 g; Sugars: 35 g; Carbohydrates: 41 g; Fiber: 4 g; Protein: 3 g

Watermelon-Mint-Matcha Smoothie

Energy Boost

Immunity Boost

Weight Loss

Makes 2 (10-ounce) servings
Prep time: 5 minutes

½ cup unsweetened coconut
water, chilled or frozen
4 cups cubed watermelon, chilled
¼ cup fresh mint leaves
1 teaspoon matcha powder
¼ cup crushed ice (optional)

Looking for a flavorful smoothie that will boost your energy without weighing you down? This smoothie has energizing flavors and lots of antioxidants, and it's super light so you won't feel stuffed after drinking it.

1. In a blender, combine the coconut water, watermelon, mint, matcha, and ice (if using). Blend until smooth, about 2 minutes, stopping the blender if needed to scrape down the sides so everything is fully incorporated.
2. Pour into two glasses and enjoy.

Simplify It! Skip the fruit prep and pick up pre-cubed watermelon in the produce aisle.

PER SERVING Calories: 117; Total Fat: 1 g; Sugars: 22 g; Carbohydrates: 28 g; Fiber: 3 g; Protein: 3 g

Vegan Matcha, Ginger, and Blueberry Smoothie

Anti-Aging
Anti-Inflammatory
Immunity Boost

Makes 2 (14-ounce) servings
Prep time: 5 minutes

2 cups unsweetened or freshly
squeezed orange juice
2 cups fresh or frozen blueberries
1 teaspoon matcha powder
1 tablespoon freshly grated
ginger or 1 teaspoon
dried ginger
¼ cup crushed ice (optional)

This vegan smoothie is packed with blueberry sweetness, tartness from the citrus, and a nice punch from the ginger. The result is a lovely balanced flavor in a smoothie as nutritious as it is tasty. It's a great way to get your antioxidants.

1. In a blender, combine the orange juice, blueberries, matcha, ginger, and ice (if using). Blend until smooth, about 2 minutes, stopping the blender if needed to scrape down the sides so everything is fully incorporated.
2. Pour into two glasses and enjoy.

Substitute It! This is delicious with mixed berries—rather than strictly blueberries—too.

PER SERVING Calories: 200; Total Fat: 1 g; Sugars: 35 g; Carbohydrates: 47 g; Fiber: 5 g; Protein: 3 g

Banana-Papaya-Matcha Energy Punch

Energy Boost

Immunity Boost

Makes 2 (12-ounce) servings
Prep time: 5 minutes

---

2 cups nondairy or dairy milk
of choice

½ cup plain, unsweetened
nondairy or dairy yogurt or
kefir of choice (store-bought
or homemade, page 70)

1 cup chopped fresh or frozen
papaya, peeled and seeded

1 frozen banana

1 teaspoon matcha powder

1 tablespoon freshly grated
turmeric or ½ teaspoon
ground turmeric

¼ cup crushed ice (optional)

Papayas have a sweet, slightly peppery flavor that blends well with the herbal character of green tea and the smooth flavor of the bananas. This energy-boosting smoothie makes a great breakfast because it will give you the energy you need to jump-start your day.

1. In a blender, combine the milk, yogurt, papaya, banana, matcha, turmeric, and ice (if using). Blend until smooth, about 2 minutes, stopping the blender if needed to scrape down the sides so everything is fully incorporated.
2. Pour into two glasses and enjoy.

Substitute It! Replace the yogurt with ½ cup of chopped, silken tofu for some added protein—it's so mild, you won't taste it!

PER SERVING Calories: 218; Total Fat: 9 g; Sugars: 16 g; Carbohydrates: 29 g; Fiber: 6 g; Protein: 56 g

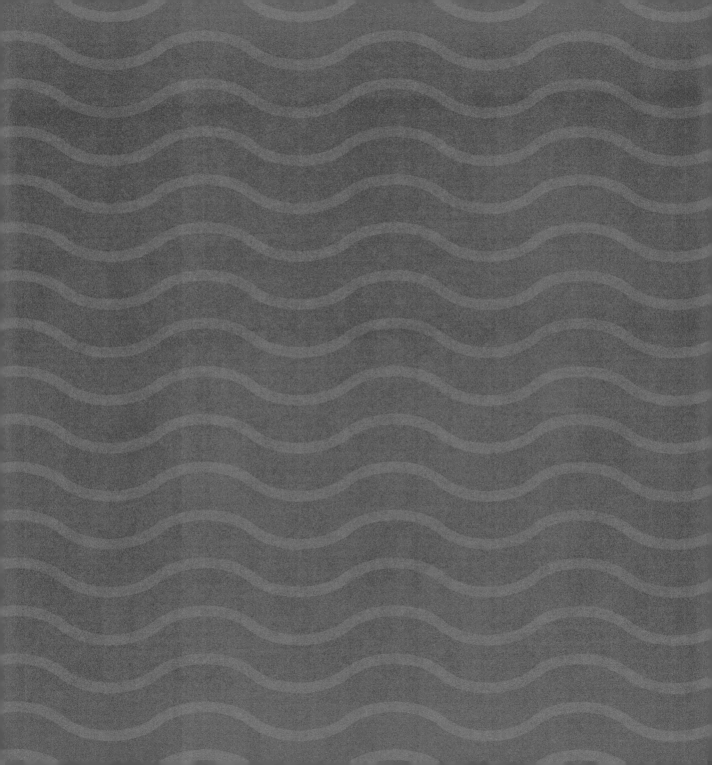

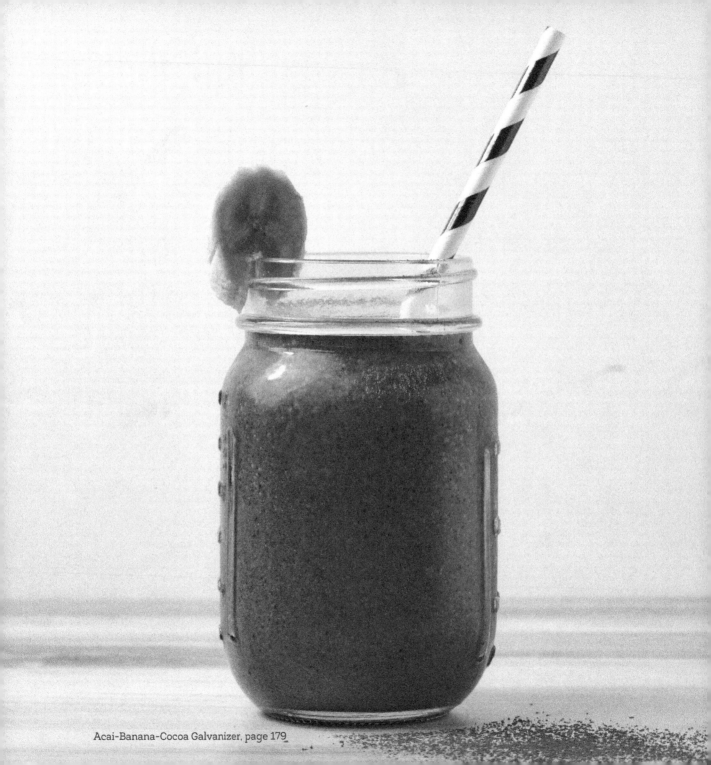

Acai-Banana-Cocoa Galvanizer, page 179

Chapter Fourteen

Pomegranate and Acai

Gorgeous in color and flavor, pomegranate and acai make an amazing duo—though I've actually paired them in this chapter for another reason: Their health benefits are strikingly similar.

Both of these fruits are extremely high in antioxidants, which, as mentioned in previous chapters, are highly effective at protecting our bodies from damage. Research indicates that these fruits are also rich in fiber and anti-inflammatory compounds—and that they have anti-cancer properties, lower blood pressure and cholesterol, enhance brain function, memory, and cognition, and aid with wound healing. Additionally, pomegranates possess compounds benefitting the reproductive system, while acai contains omega-3 fatty acids beneficial to the skin.

Acai is dark purple and has a berry-chocolate flavor (yum!), while pomegranate, depending on ripeness, can taste either tart or very sweet.

Common forms: Pomegranate is available as a whole fruit or fruit juice, and some stores have pre-seeded poms (the arils only). Acai can be found in concentrated powder, juice, and frozen purée. When buying juice, look for 100 percent pomegranate or acai juice with no added sugars.

Where to find them: Fresh pomegranate is in the produce section, and both pomegranate and acai juice will be in the juice aisle. Frozen acai will be in the freezer section, and you can find the powder at health food stores or online.

Prep tip: There are several methods for seeding a pomegranate. Try cutting it in half, then grabbing a bowl and placing the pomegranate in your hand, skin-side up, over the bowl. Whack the skin with the back of a spoon, and the arils will fall into the bowl.

Acai-Banana-Cocoa Galvanizer

Energy Boost
Immunity Boost

Makes 2 (8-ounce) servings
Prep time: 5 minutes

2 cups nondairy or dairy milk
  of choice
½ cup plain, unsweetened
  nondairy or dairy yogurt or
  kefir of choice (store-bought or
  homemade, page 70)
2 teaspoons cacao powder or
  unsweetened cocoa powder
2 frozen acai packets or ¼ cup
  acai powder
1 frozen banana
2 dates, softened in hot water,
  pitted, and finely chopped

Acai has a complex flavor that many people claim reminds them of a combination of chocolate and wine. Here, unsweetened cocoa powder brings out acai's natural chocolate flavors while providing a powerful antioxidant boost.

1. In a blender, combine the milk, yogurt, cacao, acai, banana, and dates. Blend until smooth, 2 to 3 minutes, stopping the blender if needed to scrape down the sides so everything is fully incorporated.
2. Pour into two glasses and enjoy.

✴ **Power Up!** Looking for an even greater energy boost? Add 1 teaspoon of matcha powder and ½ teaspoon of ground ginger or 2 teaspoons of freshly grated ginger.

PER SERVING Calories: 273; Total Fat: 13 g; Sugars: 17 g; Carbohydrates: 37 g; Fiber: 11 g; Protein: 11 g

Acai-Blueberry-Turmeric Smoothie

Anti-Inflammatory

Energy Boost

Greens Lover

Immunity Boost

Makes 2 (12-ounce) servings
Prep time: 5 minutes

---

2 cups unsweetened 100 percent
  cranberry juice, chilled (see tip)

1 cup chopped spinach

2 frozen acai packets or ¼ cup
  acai powder

1 cup fresh or frozen blueberries

½ teaspoon ground turmeric or
  2 teaspoons grated turmeric

¼ cup crushed ice (optional)

Soothe inflammation and give yourself an energy boost with this richly flavored sweet smoothie. The blueberries and acai have similar flavor profiles, which adds to the depth of flavor.

1. In a blender, combine the cranberry juice, spinach, acai, blueberries, turmeric, and ice (if using). Blend until smooth, about 3 minutes, stopping the blender if needed to scrape down the sides so everything is fully incorporated.
2. Pour into two glasses and enjoy.

Substitute It! If you're not a cranberry fan, you can also use 2 cups of apple juice, pear juice, or grape juice.

PER SERVING Calories: 136; Total Fat: 1 g; Sugars: 16 g; Carbohydrates: 31 g; Fiber: 2 g; Protein: 1 g

Acai and Triple Greens Smoothie

Greens Lover

Immunity Boost

Makes 2 (12-ounce) servings
Prep time: 5 minutes

2 cups unsweetened apple juice
1 cup chopped spinach
1 cup chopped kale
1 cup chopped romaine lettuce
2 frozen acai packets or ¼ cup
   acai powder
¼ cup almond butter
¼ cup crushed ice (optional)

Acai has a strong flavor that holds up well to greens. It can even mask some of their more bitter flavors for people who want the benefits of greens, but don't necessarily want to taste them. Loaded with antioxidants, fiber, and vitamins, this smoothie offers a great way to bring some greens into your life.

1. In a blender, combine the apple juice, spinach, kale, romaine, acai, almond butter, and ice (if using). Blend until smooth, about 3 minutes, stopping the blender if needed to scrape down the sides so everything is fully incorporated.

2. Pour into two glasses and enjoy.

Substitute It! Frozen spinach works well in this recipe: Substitute half a 9-ounce box for 1 cup of greens.

PER SERVING Calories: 352; Total Fat: 20 g; Sugars: 29 g; Carbohydrates: 41 g; Fiber: 2 g; Protein: 7 g

Orange, Pom, and Ginger Antioxidant Power

Anti-Inflammatory
Immunity Boost

Makes 2 (14-ounce) servings
Prep time: 5 minutes

2 cups unsweetened 100 percent
    pomegranate juice
½ cup plain, unsweetened
    nondairy or dairy yogurt or
    kefir of choice (store-bought or
    homemade, page 70)
2 oranges, peeled and sectioned
½ teaspoon ground ginger or
    1 tablespoon grated gingerroot
¼ cup hemp seeds

Like acai, pomegranate has a strong flavor, but it blends very well with the sweetness of oranges and the spiciness of ginger. With the addition of yogurt, this smoothie provides enough staying power to serve as an antioxidant-rich meal replacement.

1. In a blender, combine the pomegranate juice, yogurt, oranges, ginger, and hemp seeds. Blend until smooth, about 2 minutes, stopping the blender if needed to scrape down the sides so everything is fully incorporated.
2. Pour into two glasses and enjoy.

✳ **Power Up!** Add 1 teaspoon of matcha powder to boost antioxidants and increase your energy level.

PER SERVING Calories: 395; Total Fat: 7 g; Sugars: 52 g; Carbohydrates: 62 g; Fiber: 5 g; Protein: 7 g

Blueberry-Kale-Pom Antioxidant Kick

Anti-Inflammatory

Greens Lover

Heart Healthy

Makes 2 (12-ounce) servings
Prep time: 5 minutes

---

2 cups unsweetened 100 percent
    pomegranate juice
2 cups chopped and
    stemmed kale
1 cup fresh or frozen blueberries
1 frozen banana, peeled and
    chopped, frozen
¼ cup sunflower seed butter
¼ cup crushed ice (optional)

With a high antioxidant score from a healthy dose of blueberries and pomegranates, this sweet smoothie can stand up to the strong flavor of the kale. You'll get not only a great dose of antioxidants but also lots of fiber for heart and digestive health.

1. In a blender, combine the pomegranate juice, kale, blueberries, banana, sunflower seed butter, and ice (if using). Blend until smooth, about 3 minutes, stopping the blender if needed to scrape down the sides so everything is fully incorporated.
2. Pour into two glasses and enjoy.

✷ **Power Up!** Add 1 tablespoon freshly grated ginger or ½ teaspoon ground ginger for a pop of spice and additional nutrition.

PER SERVING Calories: 462; Total Fat: 16 g; Sugars: 46 g; Carbohydrates: 77 g; Fiber: 4 g; Protein: 10 g

Tropical Mango-Pom Energy Lift

Energy Boost

Immunity Boost

Makes 2 (14-ounce) servings
Prep time: 5 minutes

1¼ cups unsweetened
   100 percent pomegranate juice
¼ cup full-fat coconut milk
2 cups cubed fresh or
   frozen mango
¼ cup hemp seeds or
   ground almonds
¼ cup crushed ice (optional)

Give your digestion and energy levels a boost with this enzyme-rich, tropical-flavored treat. Pomegranate has a nice acidity; it isn't overly sweet, so it blends well with sweet mango and smooth coconut. If you're feeling sluggish or just a bit bloated, this smoothie is the one for you.

1. In a blender, combine the pomegranate juice, coconut milk, mango, hemp seeds, and ice (if using). Blend until smooth, about 2 minutes, stopping the blender if needed to scrape down the sides so everything is fully incorporated.
2. Pour into two glasses and enjoy.

Simplify It! Skip the hemp seeds for a simpler smoothie.

PER SERVING Calories: 494; Total Fat: 12 g; Sugars: 68 g; Carbohydrates: 77 g; Fiber: 3 g; Protein: 5 g

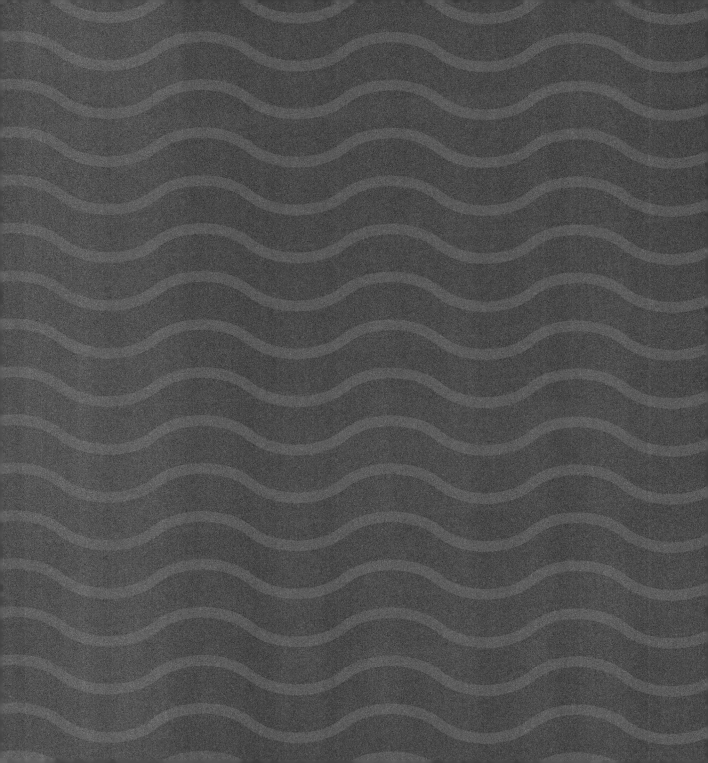

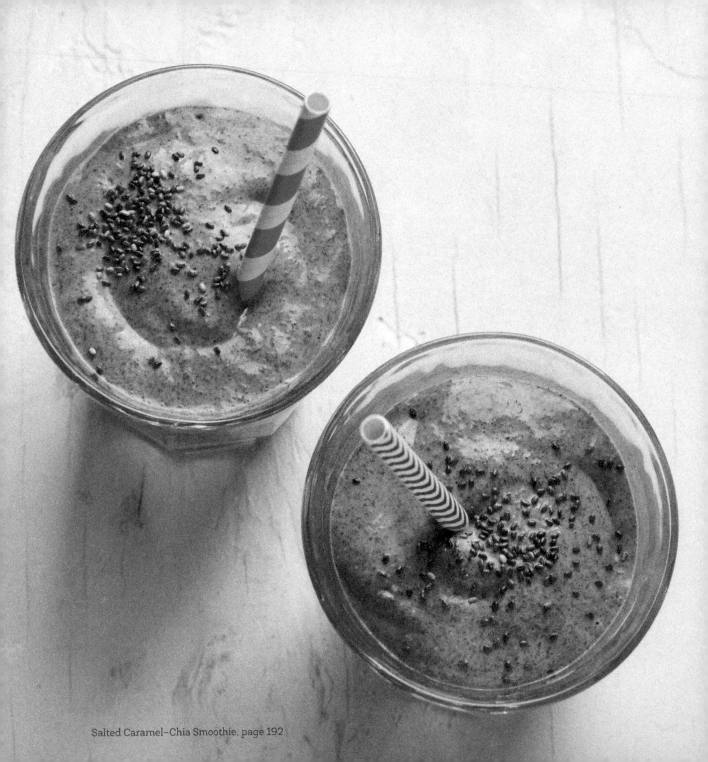

Salted Caramel–Chia Smoothie, page 192

Chapter Fifteen

Chia Seeds

Chia seeds were popular in the '80s—but not for eating. They were used to grow chia pets! Our attitude toward chia seeds has drastically changed from a jokey commercial jingle to a powerful, respected, and widely consumed superfood.

Chia seeds are the smallest superfood in this book yet are significant in nutrients, including antioxidants, fiber, protein, omega-3 fatty acids, and minerals like calcium, iron, magnesium, and zinc. These nutrients all work together to reduce inflammation throughout the body, balance blood sugar levels, encourage weight loss, support bone health, lower blood pressure and cholesterol, and enhance the immune system.

Chia seeds swell in water, creating a mucilaginous texture that is soothing to the digestive tract. This viscous texture also helps thicken smoothies, puddings, mousses, jams, and tarts, as well as function as an egg replacer in baking.

Common forms: Whole seed, ground seed, and oil forms can all be used for smoothies, depending on the consistency you enjoy. Ground seeds are easier to incorporate, especially if you have a weak blender or don't like the texture of whole seeds (they are kind of like smaller tapioca pearls).

Where to find them: At health food stores, online, and in grocery stores. Grocery stores may stock them in different places: a refrigerated case, the cereal aisle, the bulk section, or with other seeds, nuts, and grains. It's best to ask!

Prep tip: As with other nuts and seeds, the nutrients in chia seeds are sensitive to heat, light, and air. It's best to purchase them whole, store in the refrigerator, and grind them before using.

Berry-Mint-Chia Digestive Tonic

Anti-Inflammatory

Greens Lover

Meal Swap

Makes 2 (14-ounce) servings
Prep time: 5 minutes

1½ cups water or nondairy or
   dairy milk of choice
½ cup plain, unsweetened coconut yogurt or coconut kefir,
   (store-bought or homemade,
   page 70)
1 cup spinach, tightly packed
4 fresh mint sprigs, stemmed
2 cups frozen mixed berries
   of choice
¼ cup whole chia seeds or
   2 tablespoons ground

It's essential to eliminate wastes, cultivate good bacteria in the gut, and maintain colon health. To this end, every ingredient in this smoothie is fantastic for supporting healthy digestion and keeping you regular—no odd-tasting fiber supplements required!

1. In a blender, combine the water, yogurt, spinach, mint, berries, and chia seeds. Blend until smooth, about 2 minutes, stopping the blender if needed to scrape down the sides so everything is fully incorporated.
2. Pour into two glasses and enjoy.

Substitute It! For extra antioxidants, swap the water for some chilled green tea or matcha.

PER SERVING Calories: 222; Total Fat: 10 g; Sugars: 12 g; Carbohydrates: 29 g; Fiber: 13 g; Protein: 7 g

Blood Orange, Beet, and Chia Antioxidant Refresher

Anti-Aging
Anti-Inflammatory
Immunity Boost

Makes 2 (12-ounce) servings
Prep time: 5 minutes

1 cup nondairy or dairy milk
   of choice
¾ cup grated beets
2 blood oranges, peeled and
   chopped into 1-inch chunks
   (see tip)
1 frozen banana
¼ cup whole chia seeds or
   2 tablespoons ground
1 teaspoon ground cinnamon
Pinch ground turmeric (optional)

Blood oranges get their lovely pinkish-red color from the presence of anthocyanins, strong antioxidant pigments also found in berries and foods with darker hues. Here, that crimson shade melds perfectly with beets, making this a beautiful—and beautifully nutritious—antioxidant powerhouse.

1. In a blender, combine the milk, beets, oranges, banana, chia seeds, cinnamon, and turmeric (if using). Blend until smooth, about 2 minutes, stopping the blender if needed to scrape down the sides so everything is fully incorporated.
2. Pour into two glasses and enjoy.

Substitute It! If you can't find blood oranges, use another variety instead. The smoothie will taste a little sweeter.

PER SERVING Calories: 350; Total Fat: 12 g; Sugars: 30 g; Carbohydrates: 56 g; Fiber: 19 g; Protein: 9 g

Quick 'n' Easy Raspberry-Ginger-Chia Smoothie

Heart Healthy

Meal Swap

Weight Loss

Makes 2 (12-ounce) servings
Prep time: 5 minutes

1½ cups water or nondairy or dairy milk of choice

2½ cups frozen raspberries

¼ cup whole chia seeds or 2 tablespoons ground

1½ teaspoons grated fresh ginger or ¾ teaspoon ground

1 teaspoon ground cinnamon

With only a handful of ingredients in this recipe, you can have a delicious smoothie ready in minutes. This is a great one for taking it easy in the morning or just keeping meal prep simple. You can also switch up the berries based on your mood.

1. In a blender, combine the water, raspberries, chia seeds, ginger, and cinnamon. Blend until smooth, about 2 minutes, stopping the blender if needed to scrape down the sides so everything is fully incorporated.
2. Pour into two glasses and enjoy.

✳ **Power Up!** Make this a green smoothie by adding 1 to 2 cups of your favorite greens.

PER SERVING Calories: 223; Total Fat: 10 g; Sugars: 7 g; Carbohydrates: 32 g; Fiber: 20 g; Protein: 7 g

Salted Caramel–Chia Smoothie

....

Energy Boost

Makes 2 (6-ounce) servings
Prep time: 5 minutes

1 cup full-fat coconut milk or
    cashew milk
¼ cup whole chia seeds or
    2 tablespoons ground
1 frozen banana
2 tablespoons cashew butter
    or tahini
2 dates, pitted
½ teaspoon ground cinnamon
¼ teaspoon sea salt, plus more
    to taste

This velvety smoothie gains extra thickness and texture from the gelatinous chia seeds. Though the term gelatinous—basically a fancier word for goopy—doesn't *sound* all that appetizing, trust me: This one tastes great.

1. In a blender, combine the coconut milk, chia seeds, banana, cashew butter, dates, cinnamon, and salt. Blend until smooth, about 2 minutes, stopping the blender if needed to scrape down the sides so everything is fully incorporated.
2. Taste, and add more salt if necessary.
3. Pour into two glasses and enjoy.

Substitute It! If you have any leftover date paste from chapter 2's Banana Dulce de Leche (see page 29), you can use that here, as well.

PER SERVING Calories: 585; Total Fat: 45 g; Sugars: 17 g; Carbohydrates: 43 g; Fiber: 15 g; Protein: 11 g

Chocolate-Oat-Chia Invigorator

Anti-Inflammatory

Energy Boost

Meal Swap

Makes 2 (10-ounce) servings

Prep time: 5 minutes

1 cup water or nondairy or dairy milk of choice

½ cup plain, unsweetened non-dairy or dairy yogurt or kefir of choice (store-bought or home-made, page 70)

½ cup rolled oats

¼ cup cacao powder

1 frozen banana

¼ cup whole chia seeds or 2 tablespoons ground

2 tablespoons almond butter

½ teaspoon vanilla extract

Pinch salt

Part smoothie, part chia pudding, part oatmeal: This smoothie can't fully decide who it wants to be, but you'll delight in the mix of flavors and textures regardless. This is a great one to transform into a smoothie bowl—it's lovely smattered with extra toppings, or double the oats and chia for a thick, spoonable consistency.

1. In a blender, combine the water, yogurt, oats, cacao, banana, chia seeds, almond butter, vanilla, and salt. Blend until smooth, about 2 minutes, stopping the blender if needed to scrape down the sides so everything is fully incorporated.

2. Pour into two glasses and enjoy.

✳ **Power Up!** To alter the flavor profile and boost the anti-inflammatory effect, add a teaspoon of cinnamon, or swap the banana with your favorite berries.

PER SERVING Calories: 510; Total Fat: 28 g; Sugars: 13 g; Carbohydrates: 66 g; Fiber: 27 g; Protein: 23 g

Green Mango-Chia Pick-Me-Up

Anti-Inflammatory

Energy Boost

Greens Lover

Makes 2 (14-ounce) servings

Prep time: 5 minutes

1½ cups water

2 cups spinach, lightly packed

2 cups frozen mango

1 avocado, peeled and pitted

¼ cup whole chia seeds or
    2 tablespoons ground

2 tablespoons tahini

This tempting smoothie gets its thick and creamy texture from the chia seeds and avocado, which also provide a boost of nutritious fats. If you'd like to eat this with a spoon, I don't blame you: Shredded coconut and chopped cashews make great toppings!

1. In a blender, combine the water, spinach, mango, avocado, chia seeds, and tahini. Blend until smooth, about 2 minutes, stopping the blender if needed to scrape down the sides so everything is fully incorporated.
2. Pour into two glasses and enjoy.

Taste Tip: Swap a third or half of the liquid with full-fat coconut milk or plain, unsweetened coconut kefir or coconut yogurt for a thicker texture and more healthy fats.

PER SERVING Calories: 477; Total Fat: 31 g; Sugars: 23 g; Carbohydrates: 48 g; Fiber: 20 g; Protein: 11 g

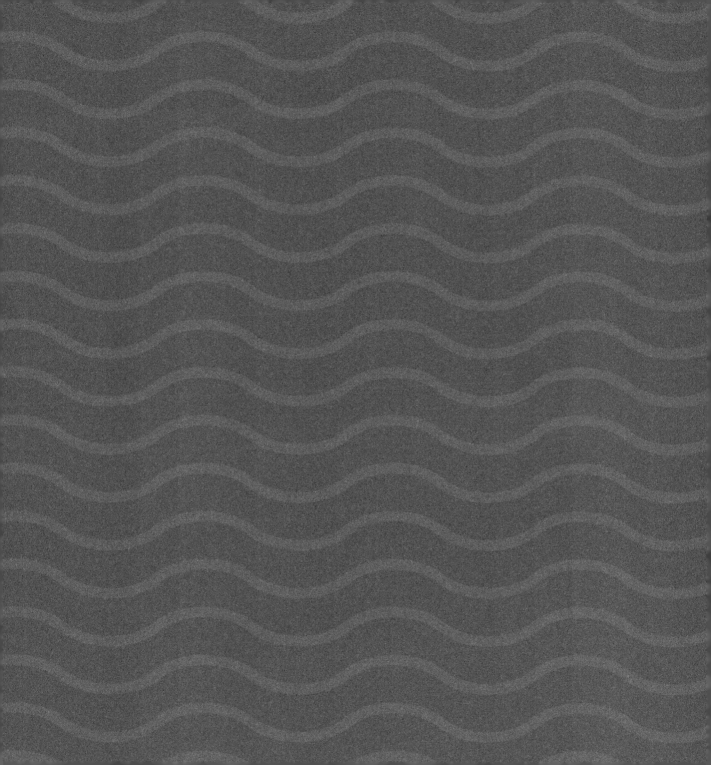

Substitutions Cheat Sheet

Ingredient	Substitution
¼ cup whole nuts or seeds	2 tablespoons nut or seed butter
¼ cup whole nuts or seeds	3 tablespoons ground nuts or seeds
1 teaspoon fresh spices	½ teaspoon dried spices
1 cup water	1 cup nut or seed milk, oat milk, rice milk, or dairy milk, if tolerated
1 cup water	1 cup chilled tea
1 cup water	¾ cup 100 percent juice
Fresh cilantro	Fresh parsley
1 cup full-fat coconut milk	1 cup plain, unsweetened coconut kefir or coconut yogurt
1 tablespoon whole or ground chia seeds	1 tablespoon whole or ground flaxseed
1 cup spinach	1 cup kale, chard, collards, arugula, or watercress
1 tablespoon freshly squeezed lemon juice	1 tablespoon freshly squeezed lime juice

Conversion Chart

Volume Equivalents (Liquid)

US Standard	US Standard (ounces)	Metric (approximate)
2 tablespoons	1 fl. oz.	30 mL
¼ cup	2 fl. oz.	60 mL
½ cup	4 fl. oz.	120 mL
1 cup	8 fl. oz.	240 mL
1½ cups	12 fl. oz.	355 mL
2 cups or 1 pint	16 fl. oz.	475 mL
4 cups or 1 quart	32 fl. oz.	1 L
1 gallon	128 fl. oz.	4 L

Volume Equivalents (Dry)

US Standard	Metric (approximate)
⅛ teaspoon	0.5 mL
¼ teaspoon	1 mL
½ teaspoon	2 mL
¾ teaspoon	4 mL
1 teaspoon	5 mL
1 tablespoon	15 mL
¼ cup	59 mL
⅓ cup	79 mL
½ cup	118 mL
⅔ cup	156 mL
¾ cup	177 mL
1 cup	235 mL
2 cups or 1 pint	475 mL
3 cups	700 mL
4 cups or 1 quart	1 L

The Dirty Dozen and the Clean Fifteen

A nonprofit environmental watchdog organization called Environmental Working Group (EWG) looks at data supplied by the US Department of Agriculture (USDA) and the Food and Drug Administration (FDA) about pesticide residues. Each year it compiles a list of the best and worst pesticide loads found in commercial crops. You can use these lists to decide which fruits and vegetables to buy organic, in order to minimize your exposure to pesticides, and which produce is considered safe enough to buy conventionally. The latter does not mean pesticide-free, though, so wash your fruits and vegetables thoroughly. The lists are updated annually, and you can find them online at EWG.org/FoodNews.

Dirty Dozen™

1. strawberries
2. spinach
3. kale
4. nectarines
5. apples
6. grapes
7. peaches
8. cherries
9. pears
10. tomatoes
11. celery
12. potatoes

†Additionally, nearly three-quarters of hot pepper samples contained pesticide residues.

Clean Fifteen™

1. avocados
2. sweet corn
3. pineapples
4. sweet peas (frozen)
5. onions
6. papayas
7. eggplants
8. asparagus
9. kiwis
10. cabbages
11. cauliflower
12. cantaloupes
13. broccoli
14. mushrooms
15. honeydew melons

Resources

There are many different places to source superfoods. I encourage you to visit local grocery stores and farmers' markets first, especially for fresh produce. That way you'll be supporting local businesses, your food will be fresher (and therefore more nutritious), and you can get to know the people who grow or provide your food. Ingredients beyond produce, like dried spices, herbs, nuts, and seeds, should be available at most grocery stores—availability and access is partially why we included them in this book. However, if you cannot find them at the market, try your local health food store or online.

Brand availability will vary depending on where you live, but here are some good brands to look out for:

Brands

- Bob's Red Mill
- Organic Traditions
- Navitas Naturals
- 365 Everyday (Whole Foods house brand)
- Cha's Organics
- Wild Tusker
- Sambazon (Acai)
- Cultures for Health

Online Sites

- Amazon (Worldwide)
- Thrive Market (USA)
- Well.ca (Canada)
- Organic Matters (Canada)

Costco is a great place to purchase organic ingredients in bulk, while Trader Joe's offers more standard-size products for excellent prices.

References

Andújar, I., M. C. Recio, R. M. Giner, and J. L. Ríos. "Cocoa Polyphenols and Their Potential Benefits for Human Health." *Oxidative Medicine and Cellular Longevity* 2012 (October 24, 2012): 1–23. doi:10.1155/2012/906252.

Asgary, Sedigheh, Shaghayeghhaghjoo Javanmard, and Aida Zarfeshany. "Potent Health Effects of Pomegranate." *Advanced Biomedical Research* 3, no. 1 (March 25, 2014): 100. doi:10.4103/2277-9175.129371.

Bassiri-Jahromi, Shahindokht. "Punica Granatum (Pomegranate) Activity in Health Promotion and Cancer Prevention." *Oncology Reviews*, January 30, 2018, 345. doi:10.4081 /oncol.2018.345.

Barański, Marcin, Dominika Średnicka-Tober, Nikolaos Volakakis, Chris Seal, Roy Sanderson, Gavin B. Stewart, Charles Benbrook, Bruno Biavati, Emilia Markellou, Charilaos Giotis, Joanna Gromadzka-Ostrowska, Ewa Rembiałkowska, Krystyna Skwarło-Sońta, Raija Tahvonen, Dagmar Janovská, Urs Niggli, Philippe Nicot, and Carlo Leifert. "Higher Antioxidant and Lower Cadmium Concentrations and Lower Incidence of Pesticide Residues in Organically Grown Crops: A Systematic Literature Review and Meta-analyses." *British Journal of Nutrition* 112, no. 5 (September 15, 2014): 794–811. doi:10.1017/s0007114514001366.

Benbrook, Charles M., Gillian Butler, Maged A. Latif, Carlo Leifert, and Donald R. Davis. "Organic Production Enhances Milk Nutritional Quality by Shifting Fatty Acid Composition: A United States–Wide, 18-Month Study." *PLoS ONE* 8, no. 12 (December 09, 2013): E82429. doi:10.1371/journal.pone.0082429.

Benbrook, Charles M., Donald R. Davis, Bradley J. Heins, Maged A. Latif, Carlo Leifert, Logan Peterman, Gillian Butler, Ole Faergeman, Silvia Abel-Caines, and Marcin Baranski. "Enhancing the Fatty Acid Profile of Milk through Forage-based Rations, with Nutrition Modeling of Diet Outcomes." *Food Science & Nutrition* 6, no. 3 (February 28, 2018): 681–700. doi:10.1002/fsn3.610.

Bodagh, Mehrnaz Nikkhah, Iradj Maleki, and Azita Hekmatdoost. "Ginger in Gastrointestinal Disorders: A Systematic Review of Clinical Trials." *Food Science & Nutrition* 7, no. 1 (November 05, 2018): 96–108. doi:10.1002/fsn3.807.

Bourrie, Benjamin C. T., Benjamin P. Willing, and Paul D. Cotter. "The Microbiota and Health Promoting Characteristics of the Fermented Beverage Kefir." *Frontiers in Microbiology* 7 (May 04, 2016). doi:10.3389/fmicb.2016.00647.

Bruner, Sondi. "The FBC Complete Guide To Nuts and Seeds." Food Bloggers of Canada. December 27, 2018. Accessed April 10, 2019. https://www.foodbloggersofcanada.com /the-fbc-complete-guide-to-nuts-and-seeds/.

Bruner, Sondi. "An Allergen-Friendly Guide to Chocolate." Food Bloggers of Canada. February 15, 2017. Accessed April 16, 2019. https://www.foodbloggersofcanada.com/an-allergen -friendly-guide-to-chocolate/.

Burton-Freeman, Britt M., Amandeep K. Sandhu, and Indika Edirisinghe. "Red Raspberries and Their Bioactive Polyphenols: Cardiometabolic and Neuronal Health Links." *Advances in Nutrition* 7, no. 1 (January 01, 2016): 44–65. doi:10.3945/an.115.009639.

Cencic, Avrelija, and Walter Chingwaru. "The Role of Functional Foods, Nutraceuticals, and Food Supplements in Intestinal Health." *Nutrients* 2, no. 6 (June 01, 2010): 611–25. doi:10.3390/nu2060611.

Chacko, Sabu M., Priya T. Thambi, Ramadasan Kuttan, and Ikuo Nishigaki. "Beneficial Effects of Green Tea: A Literature Review." *Chinese Medicine* 5, no. 1 (2010): 13. doi:10.1186/1749-8546-5-13.

Clifford, Tom, Glyn Howatson, Daniel West, and Emma Stevenson. "The Potential Benefits of Red Beetroot Supplementation in Health and Disease." *Nutrients* 7, no. 4 (April 14, 2015): 2801–822. doi:10.3390/nu7042801.

Dinstel, Roxie Rodgers, Julie Cascio, and Sonja Koukel. "The Antioxidant Level of Alaskas Wild Berries: High, Higher and Highest." *International Journal of Circumpolar Health* 72, no. 1 (August 31, 2013): 21188. doi:10.3402/ijch.v72i0.21188.

De Souza, Rávila, Raquel Schincaglia, Gustavo Pimentel, and João Mota. "Nuts and Human Health Outcomes: A Systematic Review." *Nutrients* 9, no. 12 (December 02, 2017): 1311. doi:10.3390/nu9121311.

van den Driessche, JJ, Plat J, and Mensink RP. "Effects of Superfoods on Risk Factors of Metabolic Syndrome: A Systematic Review of Human Intervention Trials." *Yearbook of Paediatric Endocrinology* 9, no. 4 (April 11, 2018): 1944–966. doi:10.1530/ey.15.12.12.

Dreher, Mark L., and Adrienne J. Davenport. "Hass Avocado Composition and Potential Health Effects." *Critical Reviews in Food Science and Nutrition* 53, no. 7 (May 2013): 738–50. doi:10.1080/10408398.2011.556759.

Fernandez, Melissa Anne, and André Marette. "Potential Health Benefits of Combining Yogurt and Fruits Based on Their Probiotic and Prebiotic Properties." *Advances in Nutrition: An International Review Journal* 8, no. 1 (January 2017): 155S–64S. doi:10.3945/an.115.011114.

Gruenwald, J., J. Freder, and N. Armbruester. "Cinnamon and Health." *Crit Rev Food Sci Nutr* 50, no. 9 (October 2010): 822–34.

"Guide to Dark Leafy Greens and How to Use Them." Academy of Culinary Nutrition. April 18, 2018. Accessed April 8, 2019. https://www.culinarynutrition.com/guide-to-dark-leafy-greens-how-to-use-them/.

Hewlings, Susan, and Douglas Kalman. "Curcumin: A Review of Its' Effects on Human Health." *Foods* 6, no. 10 (October 22, 2017): 92. doi:10.3390/foods6100092.

Khoo, Hock Eng, Azrina Azlan, Sou Teng Tang, and See Meng Lim. "Anthocyanidins and Anthocyanins: Colored Pigments as Food, Pharmaceutical Ingredients, and the Potential Health Benefits." *Food & Nutrition Research* 61, no. 1 (August 2017): 1361779. doi:10.1080/16546628.2017.1361779.

King, Margie. "6 Healthy Reasons to Eat More Real Cinnamon (Not Its Cousin)." GreenMedInfo. July 03, 2015. Accessed April 15, 2019. http://www.greenmedinfo.com/blog/6-healthy -reasons-eat-more-real-cinnamon-not-its-cousin.

Lisko, Daniel, G. Johnston, and Carl Johnston. "Effects of Dietary Yogurt on the Healthy Human Gastrointestinal (GI) Microbiome." *Microorganisms* 5, no. 1 (February 15, 2017): 6. doi:10.3390/microorganisms5010006.

Mashhadi, Nafiseh Shokri, Reza Ghiasvand, Gholamreza Askari, Mitra Hariri, Leila Darvishi, and Mohammad Reza Mofid. "Anti-Oxidative and Anti-Inflammatory Effects of Ginger in Health and Physical Activity: Review of Current Evidence." *Int J Prev Med* 4 (April 2013): S36–42.

Mckay, Diane, Misha Eliasziw, C. Chen, and Jeffrey Blumberg. "A Pecan-Rich Diet Improves Cardiometabolic Risk Factors in Overweight and Obese Adults: A Randomized Controlled Trial." *Nutrients* 10, no. 3 (March 11, 2018): 339. doi:10.3390/nu10030339.

Mie, Axel, Helle Raun Andersen, Stefan Gunnarsson, Johannes Kahl, Emmanuelle Kesse-Guyot, Ewa Rembiałkowska, Gianluca Quaglio, and Philippe Grandjean. "Human Health Implica-tions of Organic Food and Organic Agriculture: A Comprehensive Review." *Environmental Health* 16, no. 1 (October 27, 2017). doi:10.1186/s12940-017-0315-4.

Olas, Beata. "Berry Phenolic Antioxidants – Implications for Human Health?" *Frontiers in Phar-macology* 9, no. 78 (March 26, 2018). doi:10.3389/fphar.2018.00078.

Rahimi, Parisa, Saeed Abedimanesh, Seyed Alireza Mesbah-Namin, and Alireza Ostadrahimi. "Betalains, the Nature-inspired Pigments, in Health and Diseases." *Critical Reviews in Food Science and Nutrition*, May 30, 2018, 1–30. doi:10.1080/10408398.2018.1479830.

Rahmani, Arshadhusain, Mohammeda Alsahli, Salahm Aly, Masooda Khan, and Yousefh Aldebasi. "Role of Curcumin in Disease Prevention and Treatment." *Advanced Biomedical Research* 7, no. 1 (February 28, 2018): 38. doi:10.4103/abr.abr_147_16.

Rao, Pasupuleti Visweswara, and Siew Hua Gan. "Cinnamon: A Multifaceted Medicinal Plant." *Evidence-Based Complementary and Alternative Medicine* 2014 (April 10, 2014): 1–12. doi:10.1155/2014/642942.

Sang, Shengmin, and Yifang Chu. "Whole Grain Oats, More than Just a Fiber: Role of Unique Phytochemicals." *Molecular Nutrition & Food Research* 61, no. 7 (July 22, 2017): 1600715. doi:10.1002/mnfr.201600715.

Singh, Balwinder, Jatinder Pal Singh, Amritpal Kaur, and Narpinder Singh. "Bioactive Compounds in Banana and Their Associated Health Benefits – A Review." *Food Chemistry* 206 (September 1, 2016): 1–11. doi:10.1016/j.foodchem.2016.03.033.

Suzuki, Yasuo, Noriyuki Miyoshi, and Mamoru Isemura. "Health-promoting Effects of Green Tea." *Proceedings of the Japan Academy, Series B* 88, no. 3 (March 9, 2012): 88–101. doi:10.2183/pjab.88.88.

Średnicka-Tober, Dominika, Marcin Barański, Chris J. Seal, Roy Sanderson, Charles Benbrook, Håvard Steinshamn, Joanna Gromadzka-Ostrowska, Ewa Rembiałkowska, Krystyna Skwarło-Sońta, Mick Eyre, Giulio Cozzi, Mette Krogh Larsen, Teresa Jordon, Urs Niggli, Tomasz Sakowski, Philip C. Calder, Graham C. Burdge, Smaragda Sotiraki, Alexandros Stefanakis, Sokratis Stergiadis, Halil Yolcu, Eleni Chatzidimitriou, Gillian Butler, Gavin Stewart, and Carlo Leifert. "Higher PUFA and N-3 PUFA, Conjugated Linoleic Acid, α-tocopherol and Iron, but Lower Iodine and Selenium Concentrations in Organic Milk: A Systematic Literature Review and Meta- and Redundancy Analyses." *British Journal of Nutrition* 115, no. 6 (March 16, 2016): 1043–060. doi:10.1017/s0007114516000349.

"The World's Healthiest Foods." The World's Healthiest Foods. http://whfoods.org/.

"Turmeric, The Golden Spice." In *Herbal Medicine: Biomolecular and Clinical Aspects.* 2nd ed. Boca Raton, FL: CRC Press/Taylor & Francis, 2011.

Ullah, Rahman, M. Nadeem, A. Khalique, M. Imran, S. Mehmood, A. Javid, and J. Hussain. "Nutritional and Therapeutic Perspectives of Chia (Salvia Hispanica L.): A Review." *Journal*

of Food Science and Technology 53, no. 4 (October 01, 2015): 1750–758. doi:10.1007
/s13197-015-1967-0.

Yusof, Yasmin Anum Mohd. "Gingerol and Its Role in Chronic Diseases." *Advances in Experimental Medicine and Biology Drug Discovery from Mother Nature*, 2016, 177–207.
doi:10.1007/978-3-319-41342-6_8.

Recipe Label Index

Index

Acknowledgments

I believe that building health is a group activity, nourished by the wisdom, insight, knowledge, and love of those around us. I'm grateful to all the healers in my life: my husband and our dog, my mom, family members, friends, complementary medicine practitioners, mentors, teachers, chefs, physicians, fellow writers, entrepreneurs, and those I've yet to meet. Thank you for challenging me to grow, change, and be generous.

About the Author

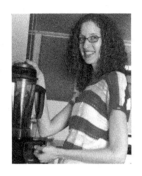

Sondi Bruner is a freelance journalist, holistic nutritionist, and food blogger who can't stop dreaming about what to create in the kitchen. On paper, she has an undergraduate degree in English literature, a master's degree in journalism, and a diploma in applied holistic nutrition. In real life, she can usually be found cooking food or eating it. Sondi knows how challenging living healthfully can be—and it's her goal to help people wade through the mud and find what works best for their lifestyles.